BREAKFAST BA...

EASY SCRUMPTIOUS EVERYDAY SOLUTIONS

(Second Edition 2020)

KAYE BAILEY

BREAKFAST BASICS OF WLS
Easy Scrumptious Everyday Solutions
Second Edition © 2020

Second Edition Breakfast Basics of WLS © 2020 by Kaye Bailey; LivingAfterWLS, LLC. All rights reserved, including the right to reproduce this book or portions thereof in any form whatsoever. For information, address LivingAfterWLS, LLC, Post Office Box 311, Evanston, Wyoming 82931.

Health Advice: The health content in Protein First is intended to inform, not prescribe, and is not meant to be a substitute for the advice and care of a qualified health-care professional. The author and publisher disclaim any liability arising directly or indirectly from the use of this book.

Nutritional Analysis: Every effort has been made to check the accuracy of the nutritional information that appears with each recipe. However, because numerous variables account for a wide range of values for certain foods, nutritive analyses in this book should be considered approximate. Different results may be obtained by using different nutrient databases and different brand-name products.

A LIVINGAFTERWLS PUBLICATION
Proudly Serving the healthy weight management and weight loss surgery community since 2005.

ISBN-13: 978-1519216090
Copyright © LivingAfterWLS
All Rights Reserved

Contents:

Contents:	3
Introduction:	5
The WLS Protein First Diet	7
Breakfast Beverages:	11
Dairy for Breakfast	43
Breakfast Basics Comfort Grains	61
Eggs: A Perfect Protein	77
Hot Skillet Meals	101
The Baked Breakfast	113
Kaye Bailey	123

WEEK OF: MEAL PLANNER

MONDAY

TUESDAY

WEDNESDAY

THURSDAY

FRIDAY

SATURDAY

SUNDAY

SHOPPING LIST:

Introduction:

BECAUSE STARTING TODAY RIGHT CHANGES EVERYTHING!

In this LivingAfterWLS Guide by Kaye Bailey, we take a highly focused look at breakfast, the most important meal of the day.

- ✶ Why is it important?
- ✶ What are the high protein options?
- ✶ What about hectic mornings?

Open up to find solutions for picky eaters; suggestions for out-of-the-breakfast-box meals featuring your favorite flavors; innovative use of last night's leftovers; attention and emphasis on fresh clean ingredients; secrets of fail-proof preparation methods for cooks of all skill levels; and comforting warm and cold breakfast meals to savor.

When you start the day with a thoughtfully prepared WLS Protein First breakfast you are committed for the day to sticking with your plan and reaching your goals.

You will find something exciting to start your day no matter your schedule, kitchen skills, or budget. This breakfast companion focuses on variety, quality ingredients, and protein options. The recipes are supported with informative articles featuring the current scientific beliefs in health, weight management, and bariatric nutrition. I invite you to go beyond the one-size-fits-all eating formulas to learn why certain ingredients and meals work to support your weight management goals. With this knowledge you can make informed choices that support your lifelong health goals.

What's in it: Specific recipes and methods to start the day –even on the run— with a healthy high protein meal that supports your goals of weight management and balanced health following all bariatric procedures. From breakfast beverages to quick-fix microwave eggs this guide is sure to please even picky eaters and take away the guesswork out of the most important meal of the day. Over 60 all-new recipes developed with the same attention to nutrition, flavor, and ease of preparation that you have come to expect from LivingAfterWLS.

Who it's for: Patients of all bariatric surgical procedures will benefit from an improved repertoire of morning recipes to support their high protein diet prescribed for weight loss and lasting weight management after surgical intervention to treat obesity.

Over 90 new favorite recipes are ready for you to try. Put something new on your plate today! Recipes are triple tested and approved by Kaye Bailey and the LivingAfterWLS extended family including bariatric patients and people with their original organic stomach. We shared these recipes with our family: you can share them with yours.

Let's power the day with a delicious breakfast!

THE WLS PROTEIN FIRST DIET

We've been told since before our weight loss surgery that we must follow a high protein diet for life. Recommendations vary from center to center on how much protein is adequate for weight loss and weight maintenance. You will generally hear anything from 70 grams a day to 100 grams a day. High protein intake is particularly important during the early days and weeks following bariatric surgery (for that matter, any other surgery or trauma) because the amino acids that are the building blocks of protein facilitate healing. As instructed many patients turn to protein drinks or protein energy bars to ensure adequate protein intake.

The Rule, Protein First, is not temporary during the initial period of weight loss. This rule is to be followed for the life of the postoperative bariatric patient who wishes to control obesity with surgery and lifestyle modification.

For most of us animal protein is our preferred dietary option on the Protein First plan. One ounce of animal or dairy protein generally provides 6 to 7 grams of protein. Vegetable protein such as soy protein has about 8 grams of protein per ounce. Sometimes getting the recommended protein is daunting, particularly considering the low-volume capacity of the gastric pouch. Often, to even meet the minimum protein intake, we must turn to modular protein supplements (protein bars, protein shakes, and protein enhanced food products such as soups, puddings, and cereals). Complicating matters, this high protein diet must be followed while observing liquid restrictions of no fluids with meals and no fluids for 30 minutes before and after meals to promote maximum satiation and nutrient absorption.

The payoff for following a rigorous high-protein diet exceeds the reading on the bathroom scale. A high protein diet helps us lose weight because protein has the highest thermic effect of any food item: it requires more energy (calories) to metabolize than it contains. That is why protein is considered a metabolism booster. Simple carbohydrates require very little energy to process thus a caloric surplus may occur resulting in stalled weight loss or weight gain in form of stored excess adipose tissue. In addition to boosting metabolism a high protein diet controls the metabolic hormones: insulin and glucagon. When these hormones are in balance, we don't have swings in blood sugar that cause energy levels to surge and then plummet. Satiation is lasting and cravings are fewer and less intense than those experienced when the diet is high in carbohydrates, particularly simple carbs.

QUICK LIST: PROTEIN SOURCES

The following is a brief list of dietary protein commonly available and relatively affordable throughout the United States and around the world. This short list provides a quick reference and is useful at times when too much repetition of the same protein has led to frustration and dietary boredom. A prompt may just be the inspiration needed to put something new on the plate. The recipes in this book provide a variety of ways to enjoy these dietary proteins.

Eggs and Dairy. Eggs. Milk, cheese, and yogurt are not only protein-rich; they also provide calcium for strong bones and a healthy heart. Remember, a chicken egg is considered perfect protein and the protein by which all other protein is measured. Low-fat or reduced fat dairy products provide the benefits of dairy with fewer calories than the full-fat versions.

Meat: Beef, Bison, Lamb, Game. The term meat is a broadly used term that includes beef, bison, lamb, and game meat. Beef is the most frequently consumed meat in the United States while lamb tops meat consumption worldwide. Bison or buffalo is becoming more readily available with the increase of agricultural bison ranches. Bison and game may be substituted for beef in most recipes. Game meat includes venison, elk, caribou, and other game mammals hunted and harvested for food. People following a high protein diet should select lean cuts of meat to reduce their intake of saturated fat.

Poultry. Chicken, Turkey and Other Poultry are popular sources of lean protein for their ease in preparation and affordability. White meat poultry contains less fat than dark meat, but dark meat protein is a better source of nutrients including B vitamins. Chicken is widely available and reasonably priced, sold as whole birds for roasting, cut chicken called "fryers", and flash-frozen boneless skinless chicken breast white meat and chicken thigh dark meat.

Pork. Fresh pork is available in a variety of cuts including chops and roasts and sold in a variety of cured forms including bacon, ham, and sausage. There is much talk about today's leaner pork thanks to improved agriculture practices. Lean cuts such as tenderloin, top loin, rib chops, and sirloin steak are 31 percent leaner than the same cuts two decades ago. Pork cooks quickly and is affordably priced.

Fish and shellfish. Perhaps the best source of lean protein combined with healthy fats, fish and shellfish support a well-planned high protein diet. Most fish contain the heart-healthy fat known as omega 3 which is shown to improve cardiovascular health and prevent the risk of stroke and heart disease.

Plant Protein. Soy, beans, legumes, vegetables. Plant based soy protein, the base ingredient for tofu, is a low-fat protein option with the added benefit of cholesterol lowering properties. Beans and legumes: High protein diets tend to be low in dietary fiber. Including beans and legumes in meals provides the benefits of plant protein and dietary fiber in one healthy ingredient that also provides vitamins and minerals. A half cup serving of beans contains nearly the same protein as 3 ounces of broiled steak.

Breakfast Beverages:

For reasons of habit, lifestyle, or even pouch moodiness a breakfast beverage is the most suitable way for many of us after surgery to begin our day with nourishment. For me, the last thing that sounds appealing on most mornings is a plate or bowl of food, especially if I think back to pre-surgery when a carb-heavy sugar-sweet breakfast of pancakes and syrup was a favorite (and all too common) treat. Over the years I've learned that in general, the WLS population agrees. A more palatable, pouch-friendly way to start the day is with a nutrient rich protein fortified beverage that can be sipped slowly as a gentle wake-up to the gastric pouch. For days when the pouch is super-sensitive or grumpy breaking the overnight fast may best be done with a warm cup of herbal tea or warm lemon water. Ginger tea is particularly effective in soothing the gastric system and it helps promote healthy digestion.

In this chapter of *Breakfast Basics* we look at a variety of breakfast beverages to suit our nutritional needs, appease our mood, and complement our various lifestyles. Remember each day is unique and what works one day may very well not be suitable the next day. Continue to explore your breakfast beverage options experiment with different products; include seasonal fruits and vegetables; and make it a habit to start your day with protein and nutrients.

Before we get to the recipes let's do a quick review of the protein basics that are essential to our ongoing weight management after surgery. After this quick refresher, we will look at inspired recipes for protein shakes, smoothies, and coffee.

Protein Basics and the Bariatric Patient

Guest article by Jacqueline Jacques, ND*

"Protein is like a mantra for most patients who have undergone weight loss surgery. Eat protein first. Eat more protein. Use protein powder. Take protein with every meal. Yet as much as it is emphasized and discussed, there are many questions that are asked by clinicians and patients alike. Questions about protein digestion, quantity, and quality, as well as ways to optimize protein intake, are very common and are important to understand in relation to postoperative nutrition.

"Proteins are one of the essential building blocks of the human body. They provide amino acids, which are a nutritional requirement of the body to produce its own proteins and a variety of nitrogen-based molecules. From the protein we eat, the body synthesizes hormones, enzymes, immune system components, structural molecules, and many more elements indispensable to human life. In addition, protein helps to maintain both fluid and acid-base balance in the body. If there is inadequate protein in the body, health inevitably suffers.

"Supplemental Proteins: A wide variety of supplemental proteins is available to consumers. These proteins range from simple, unadulterated protein powders, such as whey, egg, or soy protein, to liquid hydrolyzed collagen to bars, puddings, and cookies.

"When we look at the common proteins (whey, milk, and soy), we may notice that they are sold as two common preparations: Concentrates and isolates. There is a difference. For milk protein solids and whey protein, the filtration process that creates an isolate removes a large majority of the lactose, minerals, and fat content that are naturally occurring in the raw material. This means that isolates tend to have very little milk sugar, no fat, and provide more protein in a smaller serving size. Not always, but often, they will also have better mixability and a cleaner taste. For soy and other vegetable proteins, isolates tend to markedly improve taste and dispersion. They also remove much of the carbohydrate content. This can be very important as the carbohydrate in legumes, such as soybeans and peas, tends to cause gas in many people. As with dairy proteins, vegetable protein isolates also offer more protein per serving.

"Some proteins, usually whey or collagen, are sold in a hydrolyzed form. Hydrolysis breaks large protein molecules down into peptide fragments—thus they are partially pre-digested. Hydrolyzed protein is easier to absorb and has an advantage for patients who have a hard time digesting and absorbing other forms. They are often the preferred form for raising protein status in patients who are protein deficient."

*Shared with permission from Bariatric Times. Dr. Jacques is a naturopathic doctor with more than a decade of expertise in medical nutrition and serves as Chief Science Officer for Catalina Lifesciences LLC, in Irvine, California.

Protein Powder in the WLS Diet

It is common to see the question, "What protein powder should I use?" asked in online groups. What is surprising, to me, is the inconsistency in answers and the passion with which people believe there is only one true and correct answer to the question. It seems natural to want a one-size fits all answer and quite frankly as a WLS research journalist I would love to find that magic answer. The question of supplemental protein in the WLS diet is highly complicated and each case study is unique. I suggest that we all must find our "sweet spot" for supplemental protein intake in our diet and this will not be a one-time solution, the need for including supplemental protein will change over the years as we continuously work to be informed consumers in the quest for healthy weight management with bariatric surgery. *(I'm sorry – I really wanted to find the "easy" answer for us all, but we have learned, have we not, that WLS is never easy.)*

Here are some things to consider and questions to ask when managing your complete diet after weight loss surgery:

- Do I need to supplement my protein intake with protein beverages or protein nutrition bars?
- Has my bariatric center prescribed supplemental protein as part of my weight loss and weight management program?
- What is my current daily nutritional intake?
- Do I have food intolerances that keep me from including supplemental protein in my diet or that keep me from eating animal and vegetable protein in adequate amounts? What is the plan I have put in place with my doctor or nutritionist to address these issues?
- What is the current state of my health including age, weight, blood work, metabolic health, emotional wellness, and co-morbidities associated with obesity?
- Am I in the care of a qualified health care provider with whom I can discuss my dietary intake, specifically protein intake?

✳ Am I keeping a food journal so that I can make necessary adjustments to better manage my weight and health through nutrition?

These questions and considerations make it clear that managing our health is a big deal and we cannot leave it to chance. We cannot toss a question out for the Internet to answer and then hope for the best. Our first resource for information specific to our case must be the bariatric center –including the surgeon, nursing staff, and dietician or nutritionist—that treated our metabolic disorder called obesity. Ask specific questions of them and follow their directions above all else.

When that is not possible our next source for qualified advice should be a general care doctor, a weight management doctor, and/or weight management nutritionist. I understand as well as anyone that the conversation about obesity with a general practice doctor is nothing short of awkward. Compared with the cocoon-like warmth by which most bariatric centers embrace their patients the all-purpose doctor's office can feel cold and unsympathetic. Still, we have a responsibility as patients to honestly communicate with our doctor regarding our health. "The three main goals of doctor-patient communication are creating a good interpersonal relationship, facilitating exchange of information, and including patients in decision making," *(Nancy Longnecker, PHD, The Ochsner Journal Spring 2010)*.

Finally, we must oblige ourselves to being active in our own health management. Read product labels. Stay informed on current health practices supported by qualified research and verified studies (don't trust unsupported answers from random sources). Pay attention to our own wellness and adjustment accordingly. Follow the health care plan prescribed by our bariatric surgeon and supported by general care doctor.

Supplemental Protein Nutritional Information: Because protein beverages generally call for protein powder as a key protein ingredient the nutritional values will vary by brand and ingredients. Ideally a protein beverage should provide a minimum of 21 grams protein with 7 grams or fewer carbohydrate and 5 grams of fat or less. (With some products it may take two scoops or protein powder to achieve the needed protein intake). Remember, recipes prepared with milk, yogurt or other dairy ingredients increase the protein content of the recipe: count it all.

Stay Current: I've got your back when it comes to following the current research and recommendations for protein intake after all bariatric surgery procedures. For an in-depth study of dietary protein and weight loss surgery check out Protein First: Understanding and Living the First Rule of WLS which is Volume 3 in this LivingAfterWLS series and updated February 2020. See Kaye's author page for a current catalog of all our publications.

Kaye Bailey Amazon Page: https://www.amazon.com/-/e/B00LWITO8I

Look to the LivingAfterWLS Blog -LivingAfterWLS.blogspot.com- for current information, recipes, and tips supporting your weight loss surgery healthy weight management.

PROTEIN FIRST SHAKES, SMOOTHIES, AND COFFEE

The best part of waking up is protein in the cup! Well, that is certainly how many WLS-patients feel about their protein shakes, coffee, and smoothies. And it makes good sense to start the day with a high protein easy-to-drink meal because it satisfies morning hunger and stimulates the metabolism to burn more energy (calories) for weight loss and weight maintenance. For rushed mornings try a Ready-To-Drink (RTD) prepared protein drink. Look for a protein drink labeled low carb that has fewer than 8 grams of sugar and 12 grams of protein or more. Drink chilled or blended with ice for a milkshake-like experience.

Protein shakes can also be made in a blender or shaker cup using a base liquid such as milk, water, or coffee and adding flavoring and protein powder. Preparing protein beverages with protein powder and quality ingredients is less expensive per serving than the convenient RTD beverages. The adventurous will find countless opportunities to mix flavors and vary ingredients to prevent repetition and boredom.

Smoothies are generally iced drinks with a vegetable and/or fruit juice base with protein powder added during the blending process. And protein coffee is our favorite cup of morning Joe powered up with protein powder with flavor and sweeteners added as taste preference requires.

Caffeine confusion? For current recommendations from the medical community check out A Word on Caffeine, later in this chapter, to learn all about this plant-based stimulant that stars as the title character in many do or don't debates.

PROTEIN SHAKES AND PROTEIN COFFEE

For weight loss surgery patients, a protein shake for breakfast supports the nutritional requirements of the high protein, low carbohydrate, and low-volume diet. Mayo Clinic nutritionist Katherine Zeratsky writes that using protein shakes as meal replacements can help you lose weight. Protein-rich foods tend to provide a lasting feeling of fullness that other nutrients do not, so by loading up on protein at breakfast, you may be able to satisfy hunger for a longer with fewer calories. In a 2010 yearlong study conducted by the Department of Internal Medicine at Germany's University of Ulm, subjects with metabolic syndrome who consumed protein shakes as meal replacements achieved significant weight loss and experienced fewer complications from metabolic syndrome.

MOCHA MORNING COFFEE SMOOTHIE

Ingredients:
6 ounces water
6 ounces cold coffee
1 scoop milk chocolate protein powder
1/2 scoop vanilla protein powder
DaVinci Gourmet® *Dulce de Leche Sugar Free Syrup* to taste
4 ice cubes

Directions: Combine all ingredients in blender and blend until smooth. Enjoy at once, approximately 30 grams protein with a trace of carbohydrate.

Hint: For extra rich coffee flavor try freezing left-over coffee in ice cube trays to use in place of the ice cubes. Find DaVinci Gourmet Sugar Free Syrups online: http://www.davincigourmet.com/

Learning: See featured article, Caution: Beware of Candy Imitations, later in this chapter, to understand the implications of adding sugar free flavoring to food and beverages.

A WORD ON CAFFEINE:

According to the ASMBS (American Society for Metabolic and Bariatric Surgery) the standard advice regarding caffeine intake is to discuss your post-surgical diet with your surgeon. The following is quoted from their website page, *Life After Bariatric Surgery*.

Question: Do I need to avoid caffeine after bariatric surgery?

Answer: Caffeine fluids have been shown to be as good as any others for keeping you hydrated. Still, it is a good idea to avoid caffeine for at least the first thirty days after surgery while your stomach is extra sensitive. After that point, you can ask your surgeon or dietitian about resuming caffeine. Remember that caffeine often comes paired with sugary, high-calorie drinks, so be sure you're making wise beverage choices.

Visit ASMBS.org for more information, and remember you, your surgeon/doctor and your nutritionist, are the only people qualified to make informed decisions about your health and wellness.

Caffeine in the Diet: Caffeine is a plant based or synthetic food additive that contains no nutritional value and is used primarily as a stimulant to excite the brain and nervous system. Despite common folklore caffeine cannot cure a hangover but it will relieve a headache and provide some short-term relief from fatigue or drowsiness. The FDA does not provide RDV (Recommended Daily Value) or RDI (Recommended Daily Intake) for caffeine and the American Medical Association Council on Scientific Affairs states that moderate tea or coffee drinking is not likely to be harmful to health provided other good health habits exist.

Coffee is the favorite source of caffeine for many and one (8-ounce) cup serving averages about 100mgs. Tea may include 14-60mgs per cup; chocolate 45mgs per 1.5 ounce serving; and colas about 45mgs.

Drug Interaction: Many drugs will interact with caffeine. Talk to your health care provider about possible interactions with the medicines you take. Some research suggests that large amounts of caffeine intake may stop the absorption of calcium and may lead to thinning bones. If you are trying to cut back on caffeine, reduce your intake slowly to prevent withdrawal symptoms.

Remember! Always thoroughly read labels and monographs provided with prescription medications, vitamins, dietary supplements, and nutrient enhanced food. When in doubt please discuss your concerns with your health care provider.

"TO GO, PLEASE" PROTEIN COFFEE

We all have them: hectic mornings and no time for producing freshly made meals. Keep on had a ready-to-drink protein shake you can grab as you run out the door. Enjoy it straight up while commuting to your destination or add as creamer to coffee, iced coffee, or hot chocolate skipping regular creamer and sweetener.

CHILLED COFFEE PROTEIN SHAKE

Ingredients:
1 scoop coffee flavored protein powder (chocolate or vanilla flavor may be substituted)
1 tablespoon peanut butter
8 ounces chilled coffee
1 frozen banana, sliced

Directions: Chill coffee overnight. Add all ingredients to high speed blender and blend until smooth. Enjoy! Makes one serving. Protein content and nutritional information will vary by brand of protein powder used. See product label for nutritional information.

CAPPUCCINO COOLER

Ingredients:
1 cup black coffee, room temperature
1/4- cup half-and-half
1 scoop whey protein powder, unflavored or vanilla flavor
1-2 cups crushed ice
1 packet low-calorie sweetener (optional)

Directions: Place all ingredients in a blender and combine until smooth. Enjoy this refreshing cooler as an afternoon refresher and pick-me-up. Makes 1 serving: 150 calories; 23 grams protein; 7 grams carbohydrate; 3 grams fat.

HIGH PROTEIN COFFEE

In this example we use hot brewed coffee as the base for the protein drink. For variety hot sugar-free chocolate may also be prepared and fortified with protein powder for a warm breakfast beverage.

Ingredients:
1 scoop or 1 packet of flavored protein powder
1 cup (8 ounces) cooled black coffee (allow temperature to drop below 135°F)

Directions: Brew coffee, pour into coffee mug allowing room for protein powder. Allow coffee to cool (135°F degrees). Mix in 1 scoop or 1 packet of flavored protein powder. Depending on protein powder used, one cup of high protein coffee can provide 80-100 calories, approximately 20 grams protein.

Helpful Hint: Protein powders added to hot liquids tend to curdle and become unpalatable and they should never be boiled. Close attention to liquid temperature can prevent this problem. Most protein mixes recommend adding protein powder to warm liquid of less than 135°F. Be certain to check label instructions and use a calibrated kitchen thermometer to accurately read liquid temperature. If you are without a thermometer try this trick for making delicious protein coffee: Brew coffee as directed and enjoy the first half of the cup without protein powder. At this point add 1 scoop or pack of protein and stir until dissolved. Next, add a little additional hot coffee and stir until well blended. Finally, top the mug with hot coffee to make the desired serving size, stirring as needed.

CAUTION: BEWARE OF CANDY IMITATIONS

There is available a goodly amount of advice and instruction for making taste-alike protein drinks that imitate the flavors of candy and confections using artificial flavors and artificial sweeteners. Though tempting to use these to satisfy a sweet tooth these fake candy-like beverages may be counterproductive to our weight loss goals and healthy weight management objectives. Artificial sweeteners, like the sugar they replace, have little nutritional value and may cause unpleasant side effects including headaches, diarrhea, and increased appetite. More alarming, rather than satisfy a sweet craving they may contribute to increased sugar cravings.

Mayo Clinic experts warn against including artificial sweets in the diet in favor of natural sweets found in a variety of seasonal fruits and berries. "Many ready-to-eat foods using low-calorie sweeteners –such as diet sodas, candies and cookies—have little nutritional value and should be avoided. In addition, new studies have raised concerns that consuming foods containing low-calorie sweeteners may actually lead to increased calorie intake and weight gain." *(Mayo Clinic Diabetes Diet, 2011).*

With limited pouch space after bariatric surgery we must purposely include ingredients that provide nutrients, vitamins, and minerals to support our wellness and weight management goals. It is a slippery slope once we begin rewarding progress with candy imitators believing they do no harm because they are "sugar-free." Look for ways to make protein beverages using fruit and berries without the addition of artificial sweeteners.

Remember This: If what you are considering eating contributed to your obesity before surgery it will surely contribute to your obesity after surgery.

REFRESHER: SIMPLE SUGAR CARBOHYDRATES

Sugar falls into the carbohydrate category of food nutrition. Remember there are three nutrient categories: protein, fat, carbohydrate. Vegetables are considered the best carbohydrate source for people after weight loss surgery because they are low calorie, low in fat and sodium, and high in dietary fiber. They also provide essential minerals and health promoting phytochemicals. Fruit is also a carbohydrate that provides nutrients and adds a variety of flavor to a high protein diet.

It is important to be aware of all sugars contained in a recipe. This can be accomplished by carefully reading the recipe looking for redundant sugar such as a protein powder containing sugar or artificial sweetener and the addition of other sweet ingredients such as fruit or artificial sweetener. Avoid recipes that contain multiple sugar or sweetening ingredients. Look for these hints for the type of sugar found in food:

Natural Sugars: found in foods such as fruits, milk and milk products (yogurt and ice cream). When choosing dairy products, focus on low-fat and fat-free.

Added Sugars: Added to foods such as desserts and candy. Includes table sugar, honey, jelly, syrups and other processed sweets which are generally high in calories with little nutritional value.

Artificial or High-Intensity Sweeteners: saccharin, aspartame, acesulfame potassium (Ace-K), sucralose, neotame, and advantame High-intensity sweeteners are commonly used as sugar substitutes or sugar alternatives because they are many times sweeter than sugar but contribute only a few to no calories when added to foods. Currently six high-intensity sweeteners are FDA-approved as food additives in the United States: saccharin, aspartame, acesulfame potassium (Ace-K), sucralose, neotame, and advantame.

In 2014 the Food and Drug Administration clarified the use and labeling of high intensity sweeteners, "High-intensity sweeteners are widely used in foods and beverages marketed as sugar-free or diet, including baked goods, soft drinks, powdered drink mixes, candy, puddings, canned foods, jams and jellies, dairy products, and scores of other foods and beverages. Consumers can identify the presence of high-intensity sweeteners by name in the ingredient list on food product labels." Look for: saccharin, aspartame, acesulfame potassium (Ace-K), sucralose, neotame, and advantame.

Sugar Alcohols: this is another class of sweeteners which are used as sugar substitutes in many foods labeled safe for diabetic consumption. The FDA recognizes the following sugar alcohols identified on the ingredients list as sorbitol, xylitol, lactitol, mannitol, erythritol, and maltitol. The sweetness of sugar alcohols varies from 25% to 100% as sweet as sugar. Sugar alcohols are slightly lower in calories than sugar and do not promote tooth decay or cause a sudden increase in blood glucose. They are used primarily to sweeten sugar-free candies, cookies, and chewing gums.

Current studies suggest sugar alcohols pose few health concerns for consumers. However, when eaten in large amounts, usually more than 50 grams but sometimes as little as 10 grams, sugar alcohols can have a laxative effect, causing bloating, intestinal gas, cramping, and diarrhea. Always refer to product labeling for information and warnings about a potential laxative effect associated with sugar alcohol sweetened products. Do not exceed serving size when eating any product sweetened with sugar alcohol. Avoid free-serving sugar-alcohol sweets without awareness to portion control. Unchecked consumption can easily get out of control and the resulting digestive distress could be immediate and dramatic.

The Bottom Line on Sweets: With or without weight loss surgery for weight management the advice on including sweets in a healthy diet is the same: Use moderation in consumption and be informed when making food choices. Mayo Clinic experts suggest, "Get informed and look beyond the hype. While artificial sweeteners and sugar substitutes may help with weight management, they aren't a magic bullet and should be used only in moderation. Just because a food is marketed as sugar-free doesn't mean it's free of calories." The Mayo experts warn us, "If you eat too many sugar-free foods, you can still gain weight if they have other ingredients that contain calories."

Most importantly for us after weight loss surgery: all food choices must provide essential nutrients to compensate for low volume food intake and compromised nutritional absorption resulting from surgery.

Yummy Shakes: Try these Classic Flavors

At first glance the following two recipes may feel like "candy imitators" but look closely: the flavors come from the ingredients, not from artificial flavors or imitation ingredients.

Peanut Butter Cup Protein Shake

Satisfy that peanut butter cup craving with this easy to make protein shake and get your morning started right. I like to use one ready-to-drink shake for making ice cubes to use in place of regular ice in this tasty meal.

Ingredients:
1 ready-to-drink protein drink, chocolate
2 tablespoons smooth peanut butter
4-6 ice cubes

Directions: Place all ingredients in a blender and pulse until combined and milkshake consistency. Enjoy on your morning commute. Depending upon the ready-to-drink beverage one serving can provide up to 26 grams protein and fewer than 6 carbs for around 280 calories.

Strawberry Cheesecake Shake

The cream cheese in this shake lends a creamy texture and the use of a ready-to-drink protein drink ensures good blending and adequate protein for an appetite satisfying morning meal.

Ingredients:
2 ounces 1/3-reduced fat cream cheese, softened
1 (11-ounce) French vanilla ready-to-eat protein drink, chilled
6-8 strawberries, frozen, ready-to-eat

Directions: Place all ingredients in a blender and pulse until combined and milkshake consistency. Depending upon the ready-to-drink beverage one serving can provide up to 21 grams protein and fewer than 6 carbs for around 280 calories.

CRÈME CARAMEL SHAKE

Make use of crème caramel flavored yogurt and a chocolate ready-to-drink protein shake to make this heavenly beverage full of satiating flavor. If you are unable to find crème caramel flavored yogurt use one single-serve container of vanilla Greek yogurt and 1 tablespoon sugar free caramel syrup.

Ingredients:
1 (11-ounce) French vanilla ready-to-eat protein drink, chilled
1 (6-ounce) crème caramel flavored yogurt
1/2 cup frozen banana slices

Directions: Place all ingredients in a blender and pulse until combined and milkshake consistency. Depending upon the ready-to-drink beverage and yogurt one serving can provide up to 27 grams protein and fewer than 9 carbs for around 320 calories.

PROTEIN SMOOTHIES

Definition: A smoothie is a blended beverage made from fresh fruit (fruit smoothie) can contain chocolate, peanut butter, and other enriching ingredients. Vegetable smoothies are becoming popular with the use of home juicing machines. In addition to fruit, many smoothies include crushed ice, frozen fruit, honey, yogurt or other dairy ingredients. They have a milkshake-like consistency that is thicker than slush drinks. Smoothies are often marketed to health-conscious people, and some restaurants offer add-ins such as soymilk, whey powder, green tea, herbal supplements, or nutritional boosters.

For most Smoothie recipes weight loss surgery patients will benefit from adding protein powder to the mixture and using low-glycemic fruits and vegetables in combination with dairy protein for a balanced weight loss-promoting blended meal. Immediately after bariatric surgery avoid berries and fruit with small seeds that may lodge in the suture line from surgery causing discomfort and possible complications. Early weight loss surgery post-ops should refer to their dietary instructions for specifics regarding seeded berries and fruit in their diet.

GREEN SMOOTHIE FROM WEBMD

I have taken this base recipe from WebMD and fortified it with a scoop of vanilla protein powder which suits our high protein diet. The pear mellows the tang of the kale leaves and the citrus is aromatic and refreshing. This is a good pick-me-up, especially on warm summer afternoons.

Ingredients:
2 medium bananas, ripe, sliced (may be frozen)
1 pear, or apple; ripe, peeled if desired, chopped
2 cups kale leaves, chopped, tough stems removed
1/2 cup chilled orange juice
1/2 cup cold water
2 scoops vanilla protein powder

12 ice cubes
1 tablespoon flaxseed, ground

Directions: Place all ingredients in blender and process until smooth. Serve in chilled glasses garnished with an orange slice for a stylish flair. Leftovers can be made into freezer-pops for a frozen green smoothie at a moment's notice. Use a freezer pop mold and follow manufacturer's directions for freezing and storing frozen pops. Two servings.

BREAKFAST FRUIT SMOOTHIE

Ingredients:
1/2 cup sliced strawberries, raspberries, or peaches, fresh or frozen
1/2 cup cottage cheese
1/4 cup plain yogurt
1 scoop protein powder, vanilla or berry flavored

Directions: Place all ingredients in blender and process until smooth. Enjoy at once. Serves one, providing about 17 grams protein. If needed sweeten with a small amount of Crystal Light drink mix or your preferred beverage sweetener.

SHAMROCK SMOOTHIE

The minty creamy green Shamrock Shake was popularized by McDonald's in the 1980's as a seasonal dessert beverage served during the month of March to celebrate St. Patrick's Day. Did you enjoy this refreshing mint milkshake in days past? This recipe is flattering by imitation of the original and equally as tasty. This remake changes the nutritional profile to increase protein and healthy fat with fewer calories. In comparison the 16-ounce serving of McDonald's Shamrock Shake has 550 calories and a toxic 82 grams of sugar!

Ingredients:
1/2 medium avocado, diced
1 cup vanilla flavored ready-to-drink protein shake, well chilled
1 single serving container (150g) Dannon® Toasted Coconut Vanilla Nonfat Yogurt
DaVinci Gourmet® Creme de Menthe syrup to taste
1/4 teaspoon mint extract
8 ice cubes
1 drizzle sugar free chocolate syrup
green food coloring (optional)

Directions: Place all ingredients in blender and process until smooth. Tint with green food coloring as desired. Enjoy at once. For a festive garnish top with one coarsely chopped Andes Crème de Menthe after dinner mint (25 calories) and a fresh sprig of mint. Approximate nutrition per serving: 315 calories; 16 grams protein; 19 grams carbohydrate; 16 grams fat (8 grams monounsaturated healthy fat). Nutrition will vary based on ingredients.

TROPICAL PAPAYA PROTEIN SMOOTHIE

Make your morning shine with the fresh tropical flavor of papaya, coconut, and citrus in this vitamin and protein packed morning smoothie. Use fresh papaya to take advantage of its digestive enzymes that are known to settle grumpy tummies and improve nutrient absorption.

Papaya is an excellent source of vitamin C, vitamin A, vitamin B6, and magnesium. Some weight loss surgery patients may have an adverse reaction to the natural sugars in ripe fresh papaya. In this event, it is important to enjoy fresh papaya fruit in small amounts served with lean protein.

Ingredients:
1/2 medium papaya, peeled, seeded and chopped
juice and zest of one medium orange or tangerine
8 ounces vanilla flavored ready-to-drink protein shake
1/2 cup frozen banana slices*
1/4 teaspoon coconut extract
toasted coconut for garnish, if desired

Directions: Place chopped papaya, juice and zest from orange, protein shake, banana slices, and coconut extract in a drink blender and pulse until smooth and frothy. Serve immediately. Approximate nutrition per serving: 150 calories; 12 grams protein; 18 grams carbohydrate; 2 grams fat. Nutrition will vary based on ingredients.

Tips: This recipe provides two servings. Use the remaining papaya half sliced to enjoy with your noon meal of lean protein or make a second batch of Tropical Protein Papaya Smoothie, freeze in ice cube trays. Use smoothie cubes to blend with a vanilla flavored ready-to-drink protein shake for a healthy and refreshing energy boosting snack.

Frozen Banana Slices: Make frozen banana slices by peeling and slicing several ripe but firm bananas. Toss banana slices with lemon juice to prevent browning, place in a single layer on a parchment lined tray. Freeze for 1 hour then remove and store in a zip-close bag in the freezer. Use as called for in recipes in place of ice cubes.

CHOCOLATE BANANA SMOOTHIE

Ingredients:
1 scoop chocolate protein powder
1 cup (8 ounces) skim milk or almond milk

1 small firm banana, sliced and frozen (freeze 2 hours or overnight)

Directions: Place all ingredients in a blender and blend until smooth. Enjoy immediately. One serving provides 214 calories, 28 grams protein, 25 grams carbohydrate, 12 grams sugar. Note: to lower carbohydrates and sugar omit the banana and add 2 tablespoons sugar-free, fat-free banana pudding mix, or 1 drop banana extract.

CHOCOLATE PEANUT BUTTER BANANA SMOOTHIE

Follow the recipe above adding 1 tablespoon peanut butter to mixture before blending. Try the ever-popular Nutella® hazelnut chocolate spread in place of the peanut butter for a pleasing variation.

A DIY PROTEIN PUMPKIN SPICE MIX

In recent years, the traditional signs of autumn --falling leaves, pumpkins, straw bales and cornstalks-- have taken second place behind the ubiquitous pumpkin spice treats as the true herald of the season. The versatility of pumpkin spice provides a remarkable assortment of ways in which to enjoy the strong spicier flavors that perfectly compliment the cooler temperatures and longer nights of autumn.

For weight loss surgery patients following the high protein, low carbohydrate diet this Multi-Use DIY Pumpkin Spice Protein Mix is just the ticket for enjoying traditional autumn treats while including high quality protein as part of the weight management program.

I am delighted to share this recipe with you and hope you will take inspiration from the ways I use it to support my WLS goals to find ways it will work in your dietary plan. This recipe and method can be a springboard for your healthy and creative culinary inventions.

Traditional pumpkin spice is a blend of cinnamon, allspice, nutmeg, ginger, mace and cloves. The aromatic spices lend exotic spicy sweetness to an array of treats. In making our own protein blend featuring pumpkin spice we can adjust the spices to create a just-right flavor combination that is personally pleasing and a sumptuous indulgence.

MULTI-USE DIY PUMPKIN SPICE PROTEIN MIX

This fortified mixture provides quality protein and superb autumnal flavor to a variety of health promoting treats. This multi-use dry mix makes 28 servings (2 tablespoons dry measure) per batch of Pumpkin Spice Protein Mix. The nonfat dry milk provides valuable nutrients including calcium and vitamin D and lightens the protein powder making the Protein Mix suitable in many recipes.

Ingredients:

2 cups Pure Protein Plus French Vanilla or your favorite vanilla flavored protein powder*

1 1/2 cups Carnation Instant Nonfat Dry Milk

2 teaspoons cinnamon

1 teaspoon ground nutmeg

1/2 teaspoon ground allspice

1/2 teaspoon ground ginger

1/4 teaspoon ground mace

1 pinch ground cloves

Directions: In a large bowl whisk together all dry ingredients. Store mixture in an airtight container (I like to use recycled mason jars) in a cool dark place. Use often for best freshness and to promote improved health with increased protein intake. In humid climates the protein mixture may be refrigerated. Shake container well before using to ensure ingredients are well blended and evenly dispersed.

Nutritional Estimate: (Calculated with products specified in recipe): Per 2-Tablespoon serving: 218 calories; 8 grams protein; 6 grams carbohydrate; 1-gram dietary fiber; 0 grams fat. A good source of vitamin D, calcium, B vitamins, and electrolytes. *For best results use a protein powder that contains at least 15 grams protein and 5 or fewer grams carbohydrate per serving.

Pumpkin Spice Protein Latte

No need to go to an expensive coffee house for this treat, make it at home and indulge your comfort food craving and satisfy your nutritional requirements.

Ingredients:
1/3 cup milk*
1 Tablespoon Multi-Use DIY Pumpkin Spice Protein Mix
1 (8-ounce) cup freshly brewed coffee, unflavored

Directions: Warm milk in a large microwave safe bowl until warm (104-degrees Fahrenheit) about 20 seconds in most microwave ovens. Add protein mix to warm milk and whisk vigorously until frothy; pour into large coffee mug; add hot fresh coffee; the frothy milk will rise to the top. Garnish with a sprinkle of cinnamon or nutmeg and enjoy!

Alternative method: Blend the milk and Protein Mix in a blender or a shaker bottle until frothy. *Milk: Use skim milk, 2% milk, evaporated milk, whole milk, almond milk, or soymilk as you prefer. Avoid using fat free dairy as some dietary fat is necessary for nutrient absorption and contributes to feelings of satiation.

Protein Pumpkin Spice Iced Coffee

Craving a chilled pumpkin spice beverage? Try this delicious treat for a terrific afternoon pick-me-up. Blend 1 cup chilled coffee with 1/2 cup vanilla Greek yogurt, 1 Tablespoon Multi-Use DIY Pumpkin Spice Protein Mix, and 6-8 ice cubes until well blended. Add more ice cubes to thicken iced coffee to a milkshake consistency. (Hint: Try making left-over coffee into ice cubes. Coffee ice cubes in place of water ice cubes create a richer iced coffee beverage that is not compromised by dilution). For a special treat blend 1/2 cup vanilla Greek yogurt with 1/2 cup non-dairy topping; top iced coffee with 1/4 cup topping mix and garnish with a sprinkle of nutmeg or cinnamon.

Pumpkin Spice Protein Coffee

Delicious and nutritious protein coffee can be yours any time of day when you have on hand a batch of Multi-Use DIY Pumpkin Spice Protein Mix. Treat the protein mix like any traditional powdered coffee creamer and add the desired amount to your hot coffee, blending thoroughly.

For best results when blending protein powder with a hot beverage blend the protein powder with a small amount of the warm beverage stirring well to combine into a tempered paste. Add hot coffee to the paste stirring well and enjoy!

Healthy Tofu Smoothies

We cannot talk smoothies without mentioning tofu, that odd East Asian ingredient we either love or hate but mostly just don't understand. Tofu is derived from soymilk bean curd that is pressed and firmed into blocks. While it has a subtle flavor of its own it is more likely to take on the flavors of the ingredients with which it is prepared. Considered a health-food super star tofu is available in the refrigerated produce section in most supermarkets.

To start using tofu in your morning smoothies, just add 3 to 6 ounces of silken tofu to any of your favorite smoothie recipes per serving. Packed with 12 grams of protein in just 3 ounces, tofu is the perfect addition to any smoothie. Not only will it add the staying power of protein to your morning smoothie, it will also create a silky-smooth texture without adding the grittiness or a bitter aftertaste that many people find off-putting in protein supplements.

Caution: Recent studies identify that soy can act as a food allergen comparable to milk, eggs, peanuts, fish, and or wheat allergens. Use of soy is discouraged in people with hormone-sensitive cancers, such as breast or ovarian cancer, because of concerns soy's estrogen-like effects could stimulate cancer growth. Side effects from including soy in the diet are limited but may include bloating, nausea, gas, and constipation. Discontinue use if these side effects occur.

Try these tofu smoothie recipes provided Nasoya, Inc. makers of organic non-GMO* Tofu (http://www.nasoya.com/). Each formula provides approximately 15 grams of protein per serving along with beneficial complex carbohydrates, vitamins, minerals, and dietary fiber. The carbohydrate count will be higher than expected in a "Protein First" recipe, however, the fruit and vegetable complex carbohydrates are nutritional superfoods to benefit overall health and wellness.

*GMO stands for Genetically Modified Organism and includes any organism whose genetic material has been altered using genetic engineering techniques. There is controversy over GMOs, especially regarding their use in producing food. There is broad scientific

consensus that food on the market derived from genetically modified crops poses no greater risk than conventional food. Opponents of genetically modified food say there are unanswered questions regarding the potential long-term impact on human health from food derived from GMOs and propose mandatory labeling.

TOFU TROPICAL GREEN SMOOTHIE

Ingredients:
2 cups fresh spinach
1 cup unsweetened vanilla almond milk
1/2 banana, frozen
1 cup chopped fresh or frozen mango
1 cup chopped fresh or frozen pineapple
6 ounces silken tofu, cubed
6 ice cubes (optional)

Directions: Blend all ingredients until smooth. Drink chilled. Two servings.

CHOCOLATE TOFU BREAKFAST SHAKE

Ingredients:
3 ounces block firm tofu
1 small banana, sliced
1 1/2 tablespoons unsweetened cocoa powder
1/4 cup milk
1/2 teaspoon vanilla
1 1/2 tablespoons brown sugar
1/2 cup ice

Directions: Blend all ingredients until smooth. Drink chilled. One serving.

Soy and Healthy Weight: It has long been believed that soy products, including tofu, support healthy weight maintenance. Studies confirm that soy deserves a place at your table if you're interested in maintaining a healthy body weight. Soy provides many of the nutrients our bodies need to best manage body weight and appetite, including calcium, selenium, protein, and fiber. In short, soy is a low-fat, low-calorie, high-protein diet powerhouse.

STRAWBERRY BANANA TOFU SMOOTHIE

Ingredients:
2 cups fresh strawberries
2 small bananas, frozen, sliced
3 tablespoons honey
3/4 cup milk
6 ounces silken tofu
6 ice cubes (optional)

Directions: Blend all ingredients until smooth. Drink chilled. Two servings. This is very good with peaches or mangoes. Another option is to replace the milk with no-sugar-added apricot nectar, which produces a smooth tropical smoothie. Adjust the amount of honey to taste as some fruits will provide ample sweetness without it. And like any breakfast beverage consider the addition of protein powder for another opportunity to increase your daily protein intake.

SOOTHING MORNING TONICS

It is not uncommon, after weight loss surgery, to suffer morning nausea or hunger indifference to eating a meal first thing. While my husband can eat with gusto first thing in the morning, I am more inclined to sip my way through a cup of coffee or pot of tea to break my fast. Starting my day with a soothing tea or tonic tends to lay the foundation for a good eating day without the discomfort of a grumpy pouch.

The following teas and tonics borrow from the age-old herbal healing traditions that have survived the ages because they work. Keep these options open for when you find yourself wanting to slide into the gastronomic day slowly rather than diving in headfirst. Teas and tonics are not protein fortified so use care to include a protein meal as early in the day as you find comfortable. Remember, the simple act of eating protein is known to boost your metabolism leading to increased calorie burn, and ultimately weight loss.

About Ginger: Ginger, a root herb, is widely used to treat nausea and stomach upset as well as morning sickness and motion sickness. Mother Earth News reports ginger contains a natural chemical that is used as an ingredient in antacid, laxative, and anti-gas medications. One recent study found ginger reduced inflammation in the colon within one month. These are all very good reasons to find ways for including ginger in your health-promoting diet.

Lemon-Ginger Tonic

The lemon-ginger tonic will increase your energy and work to detoxify your stressed digestive system. In addition, this tonic has a cleansing effect on the liver, and increases the production of bile to clear any backlog in the common bile duct. Using this tonic to start the day will leave you feeling cleansed and powerful with an eagerness to take full control of your pouch.

Ingredients:
2 lemons, washed and sliced 1/2-inch thick

1/2 teaspoon freshly grated ginger
3 cups boiling water
honey or artificial sweetener to taste

Directions: In a teapot or saucepot combine lemon slices, grated ginger and boiling water. Cover let steep 10 minutes. Pour tonic through strainer to remove solids. Drink warm adding sweetener to taste. Garnish with lemon slices if desired.

LEMON-GINGER TONIC GREEN TEA

Following the recipe for Lemon-Ginger Tonic add 2-3 green tea teabags to the teapot with the lemon slices, grated ginger and boiling water and allow to steep 10 minutes. Pour tonic through strainer to remove solids. Drink warm adding sweetener to taste. Garnish with lemon slices if desired. If you have left-over tonic serve later in the day over ice for a refreshing and soothing beverage. In general, most bariatric centers include tea and tonic intake as part of the daily water intake requirement.

SIMPLE GINGER TONIC

This tonic is effective for reducing nausea, a daily symptom reported by many gastric bypass patients. To one cup of warm water add 6-7 drops freshly squeezed ginger juice (peel a small gingerroot, grate it and press it) and 1/2- teaspoon of honey. Drink on an empty stomach.

LEMON-GINGER GINSENG TEA WITH HONEY

Ginseng has a storied history as a health tonic considered a restorative and stimulant. More recent studies support this claim showing that ginseng helps regulate cholesterol and blood sugar, increase endurance, relieve fatigue, and enhance immunity. Quality ginseng tea is available loose leaf and single serving tea bags.

Ingredients:
1 bag ginseng tea (1 teaspoon tea leaves)
1 bag ginger tea (1 teaspoon tea leaves)
2 cups hot water
Squeeze fresh lemon
Honey or sweetener to taste

Directions: Steep teabags in hot water for 3 to five minutes, remove tea bags, strain if necessary, and serve in warm cups with lemon and sweetener.

Dairy for Breakfast

"Not only are dairy foods like milk, cheese, and yogurt excellent sources of protein, but they also contain valuable calcium, and many are fortified with vitamin D. Choose skim or low-fat dairy to keep bones and teeth strong and help prevent osteoporosis." - Kathleen M. Zelman, MPH, RD, LD

In 2011 the United States Department of Agriculture revamped dietary guidelines for Americans in a program called MyPlate which is designed to be a reminder for making healthier food choices. While MyPlate is a scientifically sound nutritional plan it does not necessarily fit the high protein diet prescribed for patients after bariatric surgery. However, in selecting foods that do meet the high protein diet we can refer to MyPlate for information regarding the best foods for the purpose. *(As point of interest,* MyPlate is the current preferred dietary guideline replacing the Food Pyramid introduced in 1992 and retired with the advent of MyPlate. The USDA has been publishing dietary guidelines for Americans for nearly 100 years since it first introduced "Food for Young Children" in which the focus was on "protective foods").

Dairy is a good example of MyPlate information that is of value to our high protein lifestyle. MyPlate defines dairy: "All fluid milk products and many foods made from milk are considered part of this food group. Most Dairy Group choices should be fat-free or low-fat. Foods made from milk that retain their calcium content are part of the group. Foods made from milk that have little to no calcium, such as cream cheese, cream, and butter, are not. Calcium-fortified soymilk (soy beverage) is also part of the Dairy Group." Visit: www.choosemyplate.gov

MyPlate suggests adults eat the equivalent of three cups of dairy servings each day. More specifically they define servings this way: "In general, 1 cup of milk, yogurt, or soymilk (soy beverage), 1½ ounces of natural cheese, or 2 ounces of processed cheese can be considered as 1 cup from the Dairy Group." Calcium intake is always the primary consideration when including dairy in a healthy weight management diet.

MyPlate Dairy Guidelines

Choose fat-free or low-fat milk, yogurt, and cheese. If you choose milk or yogurt that is not fat-free, or cheese that is not low-fat, the fat in the product counts against your maximum limit for "empty calories" (calories from solid fats and added sugars).

* If sweetened milk products are chosen (flavored milk, yogurt, drinkable yogurt, desserts), the added sugars also count against your maximum limit for "empty calories" (calories from solid fats and added sugars).
* For those who are lactose intolerant, smaller portions (such as 4 fluid ounces of milk) may be well tolerated. Lactose-free and lower-lactose products are available. These include lactose-reduced or lactose-free milk, yogurt, and cheese, and calcium-fortified soymilk (soy beverage).

Calcium Options for Dairy-free Diets:

- Calcium-fortified juices, cereals, breads, rice milk, or almond milk. Calcium-fortified foods and beverages may not provide the other nutrients found in dairy products. Check the labels.
- Canned fish (sardines, salmon with bones) soybeans and other soy products (tofu made with calcium sulfate, soy yogurt, tempeh), some other beans, and some leafy greens (collard and turnip greens, kale, bok choy).

Yogurt, Greek Yogurt, Cottage Cheese

These days' three soft dairy products compete for a place on our menu and most often we consider them breakfast foods: traditional yogurt, Greek yogurt, and cottage cheese. All three are good sources of protein, calcium, and vitamin D. If protein is the only nutritional consideration, then cottage cheese comes in on top providing an average of 27 grams protein per one cup serving. Greek yogurt provides 20 grams of protein while traditional yogurt provides about 12 grams per one cup. As a source of calcium regular low-fat yogurt is the winner providing 45 percent of the daily value in a serving.

Both Greek and traditional yogurt take an advantage over cottage cheese because they contain live cultures which aid the digestion of dairy products that contain lactose (dairy sugar). Experts at the National Digestive Diseases Information Clearinghouse say, "While both yogurt and cottage cheese contain lactose, the live cultures in yogurt turn lactose into lactic acid in the gut, making the dairy sugar easier to digest. The science suggests that these cultures *(which are fashionably marketed as probiotics)* may help in easing gastrointestinal conditions such as lactose intolerance, constipation, diarrhea, and possibly inflammatory bowel disease.

Let's look at the soft dairy trifecta of yogurt, Greek yogurt, and cottage cheese. The recipes are flexible and may be enjoyed using any of the three soft dairy proteins as the dairy ingredient.

TRADITIONAL YOGURT:

Traditional low-fat yogurt was long the darling of dieters until recent years when good marking and protein claims shined a spotlight on Greek yogurt making it the new favorite dairy product for diet conscious individuals. Traditional yogurt is more fluid than Greek yogurt due to less filtering and separating of the whey during processing. Consequently, it contains more sugar and less protein than Greek yogurt. An 8-ounce serving of traditional yogurt generally provides 150 calories, 3 grams fat, 11 grams protein, and 16 grams carbohydrate (about 11 grams sugar identified as "lactose" on the label).

However, don't dismiss traditional yogurt just yet. It can be a valuable source of live cultures called probiotics that aid in digestion as well as a good source of calcium, phosphorus, and potassium. Read labels carefully and avoid yogurt with added ingredients like fruit and fruit syrups that increase sugar content and calories. Go for natural flavors and select organic when available which eliminates concerns about dairy produced by cows given artificial growth hormones.

GREEK YOGURT:

Greek yogurt tops the chart for many bariatric patients for its nutritional benefits, smooth texture, availability, portability and overall good start to the day. Greek yogurt may also be called strained yogurt. The yogurt is passed through a cloth or paper filter to remove its whey (the liquid), resulting in a relatively thick consistency compared to traditional yogurt. The sour tartness remains, and lower fat varieties remain thick, richer, and creamier than conventional yogurts. Strained yogurt is also lower in sugar and carbohydrates than unstrained yogurt thus benefiting the high protein post-WLS diet.

Nutrition experts agree that Greek yogurt is tops in health benefits. "There are many yogurts on the market, and plain, nonfat Greek yogurt is a standout," says Judith Rodriguez, PhD, RD. All yogurts are excellent sources of calcium, potassium, protein, zinc, and vitamins B6 and B12. What distinguishes Greek yogurt is its thicker, creamier texture because the liquid whey is strained out. Also, it contains probiotic cultures and is lower in lactose and has twice the protein content of regular yogurts.

Rodriguez' advice to the health conscious, "Skip the extra sugar calories found in most yogurts and pump up the protein by choosing Greek yogurt." She adds that it contains twice as much protein, "which is great for weight control because it keeps you feeling full longer." Rodriguez suggests pairing the tart yogurt with the natural sweetness of fresh fruit or your favorite whole grain cereal.

Ginger Yogurt with Fruit

This 10-minute breakfast is yummy tasting and rich in vitamin C, Vitamin B, potassium and dietary fiber. The ginger adds a delicious twist to the blend of banana and yogurt. Even though it is light, it will sustain you for quite a while. Protein powder may be added to the yogurt mixture if desired.

Ingredients:
3/4 cup low-fat plain yogurt
2 large ripe bananas
2 tsp fresh ginger, grated
1 large papaya
1 cup seedless grapes
1/4 cup sliced almonds

Directions: In a blender combine the yogurt, bananas and ginger. Spoon out meat of papaya and divide papaya and grapes between two bowls. Mix with blended yogurt and top with sliced almonds.

YOGURT PARFAITS

Yogurt parfaits are popular coffee shop offerings these days for a smart dining choice away from home. But don't wait for an eating out occasion to enjoy this healthy meal, they are quite easy to make at home. Simply layer a serving of yogurt with a variety of fresh ingredients to fit the season, the meal, or even the mood. Measure wisely: The U.S. Department of Agriculture's ChooseMyPlate.gov, defines a serving of any type of yogurt, including Greek yogurt as 1 cup, or 8 fluid ounces. Weight loss surgery patients may wish to decrease the serving size to 1/2 cup of yogurt or adjust the serving in response to the volume required to achieve pouch fullness. Do not exceed the 1 cup serving size and avoid eating out of the container without measuring serving size.

Yogurt provides a good medium in which to include protein powder as a means of increasing daily protein intake. Consider adding a half-scoop of your favorite protein powder to the recipes below. For best results add protein powder to yogurt and blend well with a spoon, allow to rest 5-10 minutes before assembling and enjoying the parfait.

Enjoy these parfait combinations and use them as inspiration for your own creations. Use the following nutritional information to approximate the nutritional value in your yogurt parfait:

Traditional Plain Low-Fat Yogurt: Per 1 cup serving: 140 calories, 11 grams protein, 15 grams carbohydrate, 3.5 grams fat, 0 grams dietary fiber.

Traditional Plain Nonfat Yogurt: Per 1 cup serving: 100 calories, 11 grams protein, 15 grams carbohydrate, 0 grams fat, 0 grams dietary fiber.

Greek Nonfat Yogurt: Per 1 cup serving: 120 calories, 22 grams protein, 9 grams carbohydrate, 0 grams fat, 0 grams dietary fiber.

Traditional Greek Yogurt: Per 1 cup serving traditional Greek yogurt: 190 calories, 20 grams protein, 9 grams carbohydrate, 9 grams fat, 0 grams dietary fiber.

RED, WHITE, & BLUE BERRY PARFAIT

Ingredients:
1 cup yogurt of choice
1/2 cup blueberries
1/2 cup strawberries
1/2 cup raspberries
1 tablespoon slivered almonds

Directions: Layer yogurt and berries in a glass parfait dish, top with slivered almonds.

KEY LIME YOGURT PIE-PARFAIT

Ingredients:
1 cup yogurt of choice
zest of 1 key lime

juice of 1/2 key lime
1/4 teaspoon vanilla extract
drizzle organic honey

Directions: Blend yogurt, zest, lime juice and vanilla in a bowl. Drizzle with honey.

KIWIFRUIT-LIME YOGURT PARFAIT

Ingredients:
1 cup yogurt of choice
1 kiwifruit, sliced
1 teaspoon lime juice

Directions: Layer yogurt and kiwifruit slices, drizzle with lime juice.

OATMEAL BERRY GREEK YOGURT PARFAIT

Ingredients:
1 package high protein instant oatmeal, prepared to package directions
1/3 cup fresh berries (such as blackberries, blueberries, raspberries, or strawberries)
1/2 cup yogurt of choice
drizzle organic honey

Directions: Layer prepared warm oatmeal with berries, and yogurt in a small cereal bowl. Drizzle with honey.

COTTAGE CHEESE

Cottage cheese, the third food in our soft dairy trifecta, is perhaps the oldest cheese produced in the New World when European farmers brought the practice of cheese making to the American colonies. That early process of adding an acid to pasteurized milk to affect a separation of the milk solids from the whey is still followed today in producing cottage cheese. Considered a fresh cheese (not meant to be cured or aged to develop flavor) cottage cheese has a mild, slightly acidic flavor and a unique curd texture that tends to attract fans and foes in equal measure. Cottage cheese is high in protein and a good source of riboflavin. While a serving provides some calcium, much is lost when the curd is separated from the whey. To compensate some brands fortify cottage cheese with calcium which will be indicated on the product label.

Quality cottage cheese will contain just three ingredients: cultured skim milk, cream, and salt. Always check the expiration or "use by" date on the package to ensure freshness, cottage cheese has a short refrigeration period. Store cottage cheese in the original packaging in the refrigerator (keep the refrigerator temperature set between 38-40 degrees Fahrenheit for food safety). When ready to use, drain the whey liquid that has separated from the curds and settled on the surface or stir to combine with the curds, depending upon your preference. Discard the entire container if mold has formed on the cheese surface or if there is an unusually pungent or sour smell to the product. To include cottage cheese in a "brown bag" lunch make sure that it is properly contained and chilled: do not allow it to warm to room temperature.

Four types of cottage cheese are readily available and suited for different purposes:

Creamed Cottage Cheese is made by combining nonfat cottage cheese with a light cream dressing. Creamed cottage cheese contains at least 4 percent milkfat, comparable to whole milk.

Low-Fat Cottage Cheese is made by combining nonfat cottage cheese with light cream dressing made of 2 percent or less milkfat.

Nonfat Cottage Cheese, also called dry cottage cheese, is made from nonfat milk and contains no more than 0.5 grams milkfat per serving.

Baker's Cheese or Farmers Cheese is a specialty form of cottage cheese from which most of the liquid has been pressed. It is mild in flavor and firm enough to slice or crumble and is used primarily in cooking and baking.

Daisy* Cottage Cheese: The following recipes are provided by and shared with permission from Daisy Brand, a family owned dairy business since 1920. Visit: http://www.daisybrand.com/

CINNAMON PEACH SWIRL

Cottage cheese provides a mellow canvas upon which to present and serve fresh seasonal fruits or berries any time of the year. The addition of a mint garnish elevates this tasty delight from common breakfast food to elegant brunch entrée.

Ingredients
1 cup Daisy* Cottage Cheese
1/4 teaspoon cinnamon
1 teaspoon vanilla
1 peach
2 sprigs fresh mint

Directions: Gently stir together the cottage cheese, cinnamon and vanilla in a small bowl. Peel and slice the peach. Place half of the peaches into two dessert glasses. Top each peach layer with the cottage cheese mixture. Top each glass with remaining peaches, a sprinkle of cinnamon and a sprig of fresh mint, if desired. Serves 2 (3/4 cup per serving). One serving provides 122 calories, 15 grams protein, 12 grams carbohydrate, 3 grams fat and 1-gram dietary fiber.

Berry Breakfast Parfaits

Remember; always serve cottage cheese and the toppings well chilled.

Ingredients
2 cups Daisy* Cottage Cheese
1/2 cup low fat granola with no fruit or nuts
2 cups mixed berries such as sliced strawberries, blueberries, and raspberries
4 teaspoons chopped almonds

Directions: In four serving dishes layer 1/4 cup of cottage cheese, 1/8th of the granola, and 1/4 cup of the mixed berries. Repeat the layers in each dish. Top each parfait with 1 teaspoon of almonds. *Refrigerate the fruit mixture for 2 hours before assembling, if desired. Serves 4 (3/4 cup per serving). Each serving provides 197 calories, 16 grams protein, 25 grams carbohydrate, 5 grams fat, and 3 grams dietary fiber.

Cottage Cheese, Egg, and Ham Muffins

These tasty and nutrient packed muffins are delicious reheated. Make a batch for Sunday brunch and quickly warm a left-over muffin for a grab-and-go weekday breakfast you will feel good about enjoying.

Ingredients
3/4 cup all-purpose flour
3/4 cup whole wheat flour
3 teaspoons baking powder
1/4 teaspoon salt
3/4 cup Daisy* Cottage Cheese

2 eggs, lightly beaten
1/3 cup vegetable oil
1/4 cup milk
1/2 cup ham, finely chopped
1/2 cup Cheddar cheese, shredded
1/4 cup green onions, sliced

Directions: Mix the flours, baking powder and salt in large bowl and set aside. Mix the cottage cheese, eggs, oil and milk in another large bowl. Fold the ham, Cheddar cheese and green onions into the cottage cheese mixture. Stir the wet mixture into the dry mixture until moistened. Spray 12 nonstick muffin cups very well with nonstick spray. Fill each muffin cup 2/3 full of batter. Bake in a preheated 375°F oven 20 to 25 minutes or until the muffins are golden brown on top and toothpick inserted in center comes out clean. *The muffins can be made ahead and reheated. Makes 12 muffins: one muffin per serving. Each serving provides: 158 calories, 7 grams protein, 12 grams carbohydrate, 10 grams fat, and 1-gram dietary fiber.

OPEN-FACE FRUIT AND CHEESE OMELET

This egg and fruit omelet provides 27 grams of protein in a simple to make full flavored meal. Gentle on the stomach yet nutrient dense this meal is a stellar choice for our high protein diet any time of day. Serve with fresh seasonal berries or fruit and include it in your regular menu rotation.

Ingredients
1 teaspoon grated orange peel
1/2 cup Daisy* Cottage Cheese
2 eggs
1 tablespoon orange juice

1 teaspoon powdered sugar
1 tablespoon butter
1/4 cup fresh raspberries

Directions: In a small microwavable bowl, stir the orange peel into the cottage cheese. Microwave on high for 30 seconds or until the mixture is slightly warm. In a medium bowl, whisk or beat the eggs, orange juice and powdered sugar. Melt the butter in 8-inch nonstick sauté pan over medium-high heat. Pour in the egg mixture. Cook until set but still shiny, tilting pan and lifting edges of omelet with spatula to allow uncooked egg to flow to bottom of skillet (when the top is set, if desired, slide omelet onto plate. Turn pan upside down over omelet and flip back into pan so brown side is up). Cook another 30 seconds on other side. Slide omelet onto plate. Spoon the warm cottage cheese over omelet and top with berries. Serves 1. One omelet provides 367 calories, 27 grams protein, 13 grams carbohydrate, 23 grams fat, and 2 grams dietary fiber.

TOP THIS: SOMETHING NEW EVERY DAY

Experiment with toppings to keep your soft dairy protein fresh and exciting while managing a busy morning schedule. Try any of the following with traditional yogurt, Greek yogurt, or cottage cheese for a fun morning meal:

* Add a half-scoop of protein powder to 1 cup of soft dairy protein, mix well, and enjoy the protein-boosted breakfast.
* Top a 1-cup serving of soft dairy protein with 1/4-cup high protein granola-style breakfast cereal.

- ✳ Top a 1-cup serving of cottage cheese with 1 hard cooked egg, crumbled and 1 tablespoon bacon bits or 1 slice cooked, crumbled bacon. Other savory toppers include chopped turkey or ham, cooked ground meat or sausage.
- ✳ Make a home-style trail mix of equal parts dried cranberries and chopped nuts. Top a 1-cup serving of soft dairy protein with 2 tablespoons of mixture.
- ✳ Mix 2 cups of soft dairy protein with 1 (4-servings) package sugar free pudding mix, refrigerate until set, enjoy for a delicious dessert. Bump up the protein count by adding a scoop of protein powder with the pudding mix; stir well and chill until set.
- ✳ Chop 1/2-protein bar into small pieces, use to top a 1-cup serving of soft dairy protein in a "mock sundae" guilt-free treat.

Cheese Glossary

Cheese is a leading source of dairy protein around the world with countless varieties being produced by large manufacturers and small batch artisan cheese makers each year. In 2014 the average American consumed 34 pounds of cheese annually, mostly mozzarella and Cheddar. The following cheese glossary is a snapshot of popular cheese varieties that are commonly used in recipes and readily available at local supermarkets, specialty shops and farmer's markets. This quick reference is useful for making informed substitutions or exploring different varieties of cheese as part of your dairy protein consumption.

Nutrient values are show for a 1-ounce serving unless stated otherwise.

American Pasteurized Processed: Processed cheeses have a mild flavor, a semi-soft elastic smooth texture and account for a large share of cheese sales. 104 calories, 5 grams protein, 9 grams fat, 1-gram carbohydrate.

Asiago is aged to develop sharper flavors and produce a hard and granular texture. 130 calories, 7 grams protein, 11 grams fat, trace carbohydrate.

Cheddar: Golden and white cheddar has a rich, nutty flavor that becomes increasingly sharp with age, and a smooth, firm texture that becomes granular and crumbly with age. 113 calories, 7 grams protein, 9 grams fat, trace carbohydrate.

Cheese Curds is fresh cheese in its natural, random shape before being processed. Curds have a mild taste with a slightly rubbery texture. Per 4-ounce serving: 111 calories, 13 grams protein, 5 grams fat, 4 grams carbohydrate.

Colby: Similar in flavor to Cheddar, colby is softer, has a firm, open lacey texture and a higher moisture content. Its mild flavor compares to young cheddar. 110 calories, 7 grams protein, 9 grams fat, trace carbohydrate.

Colby-Monterey Jack also called colby-jack, is a blend of colby and monterey jack cheeses. Mild in flavor and creamy in texture, it is generally sold when it is still young. 110 calories, 7 grams protein, 7 grams fat, trace carbohydrate.

Cream Cheese: An American original, cream cheese is available plain and with sweet or savory flavors. Cream cheese is also available in a lower fat variety called neufchatel. Cream Cheese: 97 calories, 2 grams protein, 10 grams fat, 1-gram carbohydrate. Neufchatel: 97 calories, 3 grams protein, 6 grams fat, 1-gram carbohydrate.

Farmer's Cheese is a fresh cheese, similar to cottage cheese, and as a semi-soft variety cured for a shorter time. It has a slightly acidic flavor and a smooth supple composition. 50 calories, 3 grams protein, 3 grams fat, trace carbohydrate.

Gouda made with whole milk has buttery, slightly sweet flavor and smooth, creamy texture that develops complex caramel flavor and a firmer texture when aged. 101 calories, 7 grams protein, 8 grams fat, trace carbohydrate.

Havarti is a mild Danish cheese with a firm texture and buttery flavor available in plan and flavored varieties including smoked. 105 calories, 7 grams protein, 8 grams fat, trace carbohydrate.

Monterey Jack has a delicate, buttery and slightly tart flavor and a creamy, open texture that melts well. 110 calories, 7 grams protein, 7 grams fat, trace carbohydrate.

Mozzarella, the second most popular cheese on US menus, becomes stretchy or stringing from processing. Whole milk mozzarella is richer in taste and has excellent melting properties. Part skim mozzarella browns faster. Whole milk mozzarella: 85 calories, 6 grams protein, 6 grams fat, trace carbohydrate. Part skim milk mozzarella: 72 calories, 7 grams protein, 4.5 grams fat, trace carbohydrate.

Parmesan is made from part-skim milk and aged over 10 months. It has a granular texture and tastes sweet, buttery and nutty. 122 calories, 11 grams protein, 8 grams fat, 1-gram carbohydrate.

Pepper Jack with the buttery and slightly tart flavor of Monterey Jack cheese provides spicy flavor depth with the addition of hot peppers. 108 calories, 7 grams protein, 9 grams fat, trace carbohydrate.

Provolone is slightly piquant when young with a firm texture that becomes granular with age. Provolone is made with a blend of cultures providing rich complex flavors. 98 calories, 7 grams protein, 7 grams fat, trace carbohydrate.

Queso Fresco is a creamy white Mexican-style cheese with a moist soft texture and mild flavor. 80 calories, 6 grams protein, 7 grams fat, trace carbohydrate.

Ricotta: Available in nonfat to whole milk variations, ricotta has a milky, delicate, mild fresh flavor with just a hint of sweetness. 40 calories, 3 grams protein, 2 grams fat, 1-gram carbohydrate.

String Cheese is a creamy mild variety of mozzarella that forms strings when pulled. Available in individually wrapped single servings for great portability and portion control. 1 stick: 80 calories, 6 grams protein, 2 grams fat, 0 grams carbohydrate.

Swiss: This full-flavored, buttery, nutty cheese with characteristic holes is aged at least 60 days. 106 calories, 8 grams protein, 8 grams fat, 1-gram carbohydrate.

Yogurt Cheese: Tangy, made with the same cultures that are used to in yogurt with a soft to semi-firm texture. Generally stocked in the produce section at the market. 100 calories, 6 grams protein, 9 grams fat, trace carbohydrate.

BREAKFAST BASICS COMFORT GRAINS

We, collectively, go into weight loss surgery knowing that our diet after surgery will not provide sufficient nutrients for healthy body functions, thus we establish a vitamin and mineral supplement plan. It is true no matter how well planned our diet after surgery we need to take vitamin supplements to avoid deficiencies. This, however, doesn't mean that we cannot benefit from nutrient rich food such as whole grain.

"Whole grains offer a complete package of health benefits, unlike refined grains, which are stripped of valuable nutrients in the refining process," reports *The Nutrition Source* published by the Harvard T.H. Chan School of Public Health (formerly Harvard School of Public Health). *The Nutrition Source reports* that a growing body of research shows choosing whole grains and other less-processed, higher-quality sources of carbohydrates, and cutting back on refined grains, improves health in many ways.

Whole grains are made of three parts: the bran, germ, and endosperm. Nutrients including fiber, b vitamins, iron, copper, zinc, magnesium, antioxidants, and phytochemicals are contained within the three parts. Here's how they improve health:

* Bran and fiber slow the breakdown of starch into glucose—thus maintaining a steady blood sugar rather than causing sharp spikes.

- Fiber helps lower cholesterol as well as move waste through the digestive tract.
- Fiber may also help prevent the formation of small blood clots that can trigger heart attacks or strokes.
- Phytochemicals and essential minerals such as magnesium, selenium and copper found in whole grains may protect against some cancers.

The Nutrition Source advises: "Consumers should steer towards whole grain foods that are high in fiber and that have few ingredients in addition to whole grain. Moreover, eating whole grains in their whole forms—such as brown rice, barley, oats, corn, and rye—are healthy choices because they pack in the nutritional benefits of whole grains without any additional ingredients."

THE 2015-2020 DIETARY GUIDELINES FOR AMERICANS: GRAINS

The grains food group includes grains as single foods (e.g., rice, oatmeal, and popcorn), as well as products that include grains as an ingredient (e.g., breads, cereals, crackers, and pasta). Grains are either whole or refined. Whole grains (e.g., brown rice, quinoa, and oats) contain the entire kernel, including the endosperm, bran, and germ. Refined grains differ from whole grains in that the grains have been processed to remove the bran and germ, which removes dietary fiber, iron, and other nutrients.

The recommended amount of grains in the Healthy U.S.-Style Eating Pattern at the 2,000-calorie level is 6 ounce-equivalents per day. At least half of this amount should be whole grains."

While it is unlikely that WLS will meet or exceed the daily recommended servings of whole grain we can evolve ways to include more whole grains in our high protein diet. It is so important that we look at each meal as an opportunity to supply our body with nutrients that will contribute to better health and improved wellness. I hope you find some of these recipes and suggestions on your breakfast table often.

QUICK GLANCE: GRAINS

Barley: History notes barley as one of the earliest grains -a member of the grass family- cultivated for human consumption. Today it remains a leading cereal grain grown globally. In the United States, it is eclipsed by oatmeal for breakfast consumption. However, the readily available in a quick cooking form called pearled barley is chewy and flavorful addition to soups and grain salads. A ½-cup serving of cooked pearled barley provides 96 calories, 2 grams protein, 22 grams complex carbohydrate, and trace fat.

Bulgur: A cereal grain made of the groats of several wheat species, must often durum wheat. Bulgur is more common in European, Middle Eastern, and Indian cuisine and not often consumed as a breakfast grain in the United States. It is more often an ingredient used for stuffing, casserole and pilaf, stew and soup. The fine grain bulgur is used in tabbouleh. A ½-cup serving of cooked bulgur provides 76 calories, 3 grams protein, 17 grams complex carbohydrate, and trace fat.

Quinoa: Considered a more complete protein, containing all the essential amino acids, than other grains quinoa is a seed derived from a plant in the spinach and chard family. Naturally low in cholesterol and sodium, quinoa is also a good source of magnesium, phosphorus and manganese. Once reserved for extreme vegetarian dishes quinoa has become more popular in the traditional diets of those seeking a quality vegetable protein. Its growing popularity was acknowledged when the Food and Agricultural Organization of the United Nations declared 2013 "The International Year of the Quinoa.". The flattened, oval grain is available in white, pale gold, black and red varieties in the rice and grain aisle. The mild, slightly nutty flavor and fluffy texture of quinoa provides a congenial host for many flavors. A ½-cup serving of quinoa contains 110 calories, 4 grams protein, 2 grams fat, 20 grams carbohydrate.

George Mateljan of The World's Healthiest Foods instructs, "To cook the quinoa, add one part of the grain to two parts liquid in a saucepan. After the mixture is brought to a boil, reduce the heat to simmer and cover. One cup of quinoa cooked in this method usually takes 15 minutes to prepare. When cooking is complete, you will notice that the grains have become translucent, and the white germ has partially detached itself, appearing like a white-spiraled tail. If you desire the quinoa to have a nuttier flavor, you can dry roast it before cooking; to dry roast, place it in a skillet over medium-low heat and stir constantly for five minutes."

GRAIN AND EGGS QUICK BREAKFAST

We know that grains are good for us and we know our WLS diet is high protein low carbohydrate. To increase our healthy carbohydrate intake with whole grains is challenging. Leave it to the simple perfect protein –*the egg*—to save the plate. Try some of these non-traditional breakfast meals for a healthy start to the day that will keep hunger away.

THREE-GRAIN CASSEROLE

This oven-baked casserole is a perfectly suited medium for our grain and eggs quick breakfast meals that can be made in minutes. The recipe directs the casserole be baked in a large casserole dish. It can also be divided among 12 muffin cups and baked for ready-to-eat individual portions. Experiment with different vegetables for nutritional variety and flavor excitement.

Ingredients:
4 medium carrots, peeled and thinly sliced
2 ribs celery, thinly sliced
1 medium red bell pepper, seeded, small dice
1 medium sweet onion, peeled, small dice
1 tablespoon butter or olive oil
1 cup quick-cooking barley
1 cup quick cooking oats
½ cup bulgur
Salt and pepper
3 cups reduced sodium chicken broth or vegetable broth
1 cup Cheddar cheese, shredded

Directions: Heat oven to 350°F. Spray a 13 x 9 x 2-inch baking dish or a 12-cup muffin tin with cooking spray, set aside. In a medium skillet heat the butter or olive oil over medium high, add the carrots, celery, bell pepper, and sweet onion and cook and stir until soft and translucent, about 5 minutes. Remove from heat, stir in barley, oats, and bulgur to combine, season with salt and pepper, transfer to the prepared baking dish. Add vegetable broth. Cover and bake 50-55 minutes or until grains have absorbed liquid and are tender. Remove cover, spread cheese evenly over casserole, bake 4 to 6 minutes to melt cheese. Allow to cool slightly before serving. Use as a side dish to protein or as the grain platform for Grain and Eggs Quick Breakfast. Each ¾-cup serving provides 226 calories, 12 grams protein, 5 grams fat, 38 grams complex carbohydrates from vegetables and grains.

Note: If casserole seems to be too dry during baking add additional broth ½-cup at a time.

VEGETABLE QUINOA

This basic vegetable and grain dish can be easily changed to suit the mood or the season. Use any pleasing combination of vegetables making sure there are 2 – 2 ½ cups vegetable to 1 cup uncooked quinoa. Use hot sauce, chutney, or salsa to garnish vegetable quinoa which can be served as a chilled salad or warm side dish. Double the batch to provide several servings; this salad keeps 6 days refrigerated.

Ingredients:
1 teaspoon olive oil
1 medium onion, chopped
1 medium carrot, chopped
1 medium zucchini, chopped
4-ounces button mushrooms, chopped
2 cups reduced sodium chicken or vegetable broth
¼ cup water
½ teaspoon salt
1 cup quinoa, rinsed
1 medium tomato, seeded and diced

Directions: In a medium saucepan set on medium-high heat cook the onion, carrot and zucchini in olive oil until just tender, add mushrooms and cook 2-3 minutes more. Stir in broth and water: bring to boil. Add quinoa; return to boil. Reduce heat; cover and simmer for 15 minutes and all liquid is absorbed, and quinoa is tender. Remove from the heat, all to stand 5 minutes, fluff and serve. Garnish with diced tomato. Excellent as a side dish to protein or as the grain platform for Grain and Eggs Quick Breakfast. A ¾-cup serving provides 198 calories, 8 grams protein, 4 grams fat, 38 grams complex carbohydrates from vegetables and grains.

Bulgur Porridge with Apples and Walnuts

Introduction
Ingredients:
1 cup uncooked bulgur
1 cup pure apple juice
1 cup water
½ teaspoon salt
1 medium tart apple, cored, peeled and diced
¼ cup chopped walnuts, toasted

Directions: In a large saucepan, combine bulgur, apple juice, water, and salt. Bring to a boil over high heat; reduce heat; cover and simmer 15-20 minutes until liquid is absorbed. Remove from heat. Add diced apple; stir to combine. Serve topped with toasted walnuts.

Healthy Eating Includes Oatmeal

Every November the American Heart Association invites us to participate in National Eating Healthy Day. On this day, Americans are encouraged to commit to healthier eating. Since working in the weight loss surgery community, I have repeatedly been impressed how weight loss surgery patients not only commit to the dietary and lifestyle changes of weight loss surgery, but also resolve to live with a higher focus on health and wellness. Participating in National Eating Healthy Day seems a natural fit for our unique community. Quaker Oats is a leading sponsor of National Eating Healthy Day and they have generously shared this information with us.

Long revered as a nutritional powerhouse, oatmeal is a health promoting platform for adding whole grain to our diet because it lends itself to a variety ingredients and flavors that boost protein and enhance the eating experience. In the recipe below, Egg-White Whipped Vanilla Oatmeal provided by Quaker Oats, we add 14 grams protein per serving by whipping and cooking egg whites right into the oatmeal. The meal is further protein fortified with a topping of Greek yogurt rounding out this healthy breakfast with a whopping 22 grams protein. Once the technique of adding egg white in the final cooking step is mastered, we can experiment with all manner of toppings to please the taste buds and meet our WLS nutritional needs.

Key Point: Oatmeal, with its soft comforting texture, is sometimes mistakenly considered a "WLS Slider Food". It is not. Remember, the basic definition of slider food is a non-nutritional simple carbohydrate, usually consumed out-of-hand, in unchecked measure in response to stimuli other than hunger.

OATMEAL OPTIONS DEFINED

These definitions are provided by Quaker Oats four varieties of oats that are readily available and budget friendly. The definitions apply to other brands and store labels on oats. Please note:

"All the types are equally nutritious because they supply all parts of the oat grain including the bran, endosperm and germ. It's the different size and shape of the oats that affects the cooking time and texture. Additionally, many varieties are fortified with vitamins, minerals and flavoring."

Quaker® Old Fashioned Oats are whole oats that are rolled to flatten them. Sometimes referred to as "raw".

Quick Quaker® Oats are made the same way but are simply cut into slightly smaller pieces so they cook faster.

Steel Cut Oats are whole oats that have not been rolled into flakes. Instead, they are cut approximately into thirds. Cooking time is 30 minutes and the texture heartier than rolled oats. Steel Cut Oats are also known as Scotch Oats, Pinhead Oats (in Great Britain because they resemble the size and shape of the head of a large pin) and Irish Oats.

Instant Quaker® Oats use the exact same oats, only they are rolled a little bit thinner and cut finer so that they cook very quickly.

*The recipes provided by Quaker Oats for publication in Breakfast Basics of WLS include the specific variety of Quaker Oats found to produce the best result in the recipe. Exchanging one variety of oats for another may produce different results and alter cooking time but will not ruin the recipe.

Egg-White Whipped Vanilla Oatmeal

Recipes provided by Quaker® Oats

Ingredients:
3/4 cup Quaker® Oats, Quick or Old Fashioned*
1-1/2 cups water
4 egg whites, beaten with a fork until frothy
1/2 tablespoon salted butter
1/2 teaspoon pure vanilla extract

Toppings:

1/2 cup Greek yogurt
1/3 cup sliced bananas
1/3 cup walnuts

1/4 cup dried cranberries

Directions: Begin cooking oats as usual on the stovetop. After the oats have absorbed most of the water, pour in egg whites and vanilla and whip vigorously with a fork until mixture is well blended. Raise the heat to medium and stir in the butter. Continue to cook for 4 more minutes, bringing oats back to a simmer and stirring frequently. When all the water is absorbed and the egg whites have caused the oats to puff and appear creamy, cover the pot and remove from the heat. Let the oats sit, covered, for 5 minutes. Stir oatmeal, add toppings, and enjoy!

Nutrition Note: WLS patients will need to adjust the serving size to give you pouch fullness stopping before the discomfort of excessive fullness occurs. Overeating can occur before we realize it when enjoying a warm soft food such as oatmeal. But remember, this does not make oatmeal a WLS-Slider Foods. The basic definition of slider food is that it is empty or non-nutritional and consumed unmeasured or mindlessly. Use this information only as an estimate of the nutritional values in your warm delicious bowl of oatmeal:

One single-serve pouch of Quaker Instant Oatmeal provides 160 calories, 4 grams protein, 33 grams carbohydrate, 2 grams fat. Two egg whites provide 34 calories, 7 grams protein, trace amounts of carbohydrate and fat. a 1/2-cup serving of non-fat Greek Yogurt provides 60 calories, 11 grams protein, and 5 grams carbohydrate.

PUMPKIN CHEESECAKE OATMEAL

Ingredients:
1/2 cup Quaker® Oats, Quick or Old Fashioned* (or try 1/4 cup Quaker® Steel Cut Oats)
1/4 cup Canned pumpkin puree

2 teaspoons brown sugar
2 teaspoons pumpkin spice
1 teaspoons vanilla extract
2 tablespoons graham crackers, crumbled
1 tablespoons whipped cream cheese
1 tablespoons chopped pecans

Directions: Prepare oatmeal as usual. Stir in pumpkin puree, brown sugar, pumpkin spice, and vanilla. Top with crumbled graham crackers, a dollop of whipped cream cheese, and sprinkle with chopped pecans.

PB&J and Apple Oatmeal

Ingredients:
1/2 cup Quaker® Oats, Quick or Old Fashioned* (or try 1/4 cup Quaker® Steel Cut Oats)
1 small fresh apple, diced
1 tablespoon peanut butter or almond butter
1 tablespoon strawberry jelly

Directions: Prepare oatmeal as usual, add toppings and enjoy! For additional topping ideas, try adding fresh strawberries, honey, or dry roasted peanuts.

Oat Snack Cakes

Provided by ChooseMyPlate, a service of the U.S. Department of Agriculture. ChooseMyPlate.gov

These oat snack cakes are full of whole grains and flavor, making them perfect for sharing with friends and family. They store well in the freezer. Pair a single oat cake with a hard-cooked egg and orange sections for a balanced breakfast.

Ingredients
6 cup old fashioned oats
2 cup whole wheat flour
1 cup all-purpose flour
1 cup sugar
1 teaspoon baking soda
1/2 teaspoon salt
1 teaspoon cinnamon
3/4 cup margarine, room temperature
1/2 cup vegetable oil
2 teaspoon vanilla flavoring
2 egg whites, beaten
1 tablespoon water
1 cup raisins

Directions: Preheat oven to 375°F. Mix oatmeal, flour, sugar, baking soda, salt and cinnamon in a large bowl. Cut in margarine until mixture resembles coarse meal. Combine oil, vanilla, egg whites, and water. Stir into dry ingredients and raisins, mixing only until it holds together. Wash hands thoroughly, then dip in cornmeal or flour. Pinch off pieces of dough and form into balls about 1 inch in diameter. Place balls on baking pan (sprayed with non-stick cooking spray) and press out slightly to about 1/4 inch in thickness. Bake 15-20 minutes or until lightly browned. Cool, then store in an airtight container.

Makes 60 cakes. Nutrients per 1 cake: 109 calories, 2 grams protein, 5 grams fat, 15 grams carbohydrate (1-gram dietary fiber, 5 grams sugar).

SAVORY OATMEAL EGG, TURKEY BACON & PARMESAN

Ingredients:
1/2 cup Quaker® Oats Quick or Old Fashioned*

1 egg
2 slices turkey bacon strips
2 tablespoons shaved parmesan cheese
1 tablespoon sliced scallions
1 tablespoon French fried onions

Directions: Prepare oatmeal as usual and set aside. Coat a small nonstick pan with cooking spray and turn on medium heat. Add bacon, cook until browned, and then remove. In the same pan, cook egg until the white is set and the yolk is still runny (about 3-4 minutes). Top oatmeal with the egg, bacon, parmesan cheese, scallions, fried onions, and salt & pepper. *Can also be made with 1/4 cup Quaker Steel Cut Oats.

HIGH PROTEIN OVERNIGHT YOGURT OATMEAL

This clever method for setting for preparing a hearty protein enriched breakfast the night before is a guaranteed way to start the morning on a healthy protein first foot. The base recipe includes yogurt, oatmeal, protein powder, and chia seed. The oatmeal is enhanced with the addition of fruit, nuts, and sweetener for a variety of appealing flavors and textures.

OVERNIGHT YOGURT OATMEAL: BASE RECIPE

Ingredients:
1 (6-ounce) container yogurt
1 (1-ounce) packet instant oatmeal
1 scoop protein powder of choice
1 teaspoon chia seed

Directions: At least 8 hours before serving combine the yogurt, oatmeal, protein powder and chia seed in a bowl. Transfer to a container with a tight-fitting lid; refrigerate for at least 8 hours but no longer than three days. Enjoy chilled oatmeal with any of the following toppings or a topping of your choice.

OVERNIGHT YOGURT OATMEAL: TOPPINGS

* *Peanut Butter and Banana:* To base recipe stir in 2 tablespoons peanut butter. Top with 1/2 banana, sliced.
* *Peanut Butter and Jam:* To base recipe stir in 2 tablespoons peanut butter. Swirl in 1 teaspoon no-sugar-added jam or jelly.
* *Almond and Honey:* To base recipe stir in 1/4 cup sliced toasted almonds. Drizzle with honey.
* *Berries and Cream:* Top base recipe with 1/4 cup fresh seasonal berries and 1 tablespoon non-dairy whipped cream or 1/4 cup half-and-half.
* *Cranberry and Walnuts:* Top base recipe with 1/4 cup fresh cranberries or 2 tablespoons dried cranberries and 2 tablespoons chopped walnuts.
* *Maple Apples:* Top base recipe with 1/4 cup chopped fresh apples and drizzle with 1-2 tablespoons pure maple syrup.

AUTUMN PUMPKIN OATMEAL

For a more traditional oatmeal recipe try this fall favorite using the DIY Pumpkin Spice Protein Mix, recipe on page xx.

Ingredients:
1 (.98 ounce) packet instant oatmeal
1/3 cup 100% Pure Pumpkin
2/3 cup milk or water, room temperature

2 tablespoon Multi-Use DIY Pumpkin Spice Protein Mix
1-2 tablespoons crunchy granola with vanilla and butterscotch chips

Directions: In a microwave-safe bowl stir together instant oatmeal, pumpkin, and milk. Microwave 1 to 2 minutes on High, stir again. Allow to cool slightly. Stir in the Protein Mix and top oatmeal with crunchy granola. Add additional milk to taste and enjoy your hearty Autumn Pumpkin Oatmeal.

CINNAMON VANILLA GRANOLA

Provided by ChooseMyPlate, a service of the U.S. Department of Agriculture. ChooseMyPlate.gov

If you've never made homemade granola, you might be surprised at how a few simple ingredients like oatmeal and honey turn into a tasty, satisfying, whole-grain snack! This satisfying granola goes well layered into the Yogurt Parfaits. (See the Dairy for Breakfast chapter).

Ingredients
2 tablespoon honey
1/2 cup water
2 tablespoon vegetable oil
4 cup uncooked rolled oats
1 teaspoon vanilla extract
1 teaspoon cinnamon
1/4 teaspoon salt

Directions: Preheat oven to 275°F. Mix honey, water, vegetable oil, vanilla extract, cinnamon, and salt in a large bowl. Stir in oats; mix well. Spread mixture on a cookie sheet, making a thin layer. Bake for 20 minutes. Remove from oven, stir mixture well and return to oven. Bake 20 more minutes and stir as before. Bake 5-20 more minutes, until granola is golden brown. Break into small pieces with spatula. Cool and then store in a covered container. Nutrients per 1/2-cup serving: 201 calories, 5 grams protein, 7 grams fat, 30 grams carbohydrate (4 grams dietary fiber, 5 grams total sugars). A good source of potassium and calcium.

EGGS: A PERFECT PROTEIN

"A recent scientific study shows that eating eggs for breakfast can help overweight dieters lose more weight, lower their body mass index and shrink their waist more than people who eat a bagel breakfast of equal calories. This study supports previous research, published in the Journal of the American College of Nutrition, which showed that people who ate eggs for breakfast felt more satisfied and ate fewer calories at the following meal."

Egg Nutrition Center: visit http://www.eggnutritioncenter.org/

CHOLESTEROL, HEART DISEASE, AND EGGS

For the last half of the 20th century Americans were warned and believed that consumption of eggs contributed to the risk of developing coronary heart disease. This was based on the observation that eggs contain dietary cholesterol which some experiments showed increases serum cholesterol and leads to the onset of coronary heart disease. However, current findings have led scientists and the government to back-track on those conclusions stating that studies do not support the belief that egg consumption is a risk factor for coronary disease.

As reported in the Journal of the American College of Nutrition S.B. Kritchevsky of the Wake Forest University School of Medicine states, "Within the nutritional community there is a growing appreciation that health derives from an overall pattern of diet rather than from the avoidance of particular foods, and there has been a shift in the tone in recent dietary recommendations away from "avoidance" messages to ones that promote healthy eating patterns. The most recent American Heart Association guidelines no longer include a recommendation to limit egg consumption but recommend the adoption of eating practices associated with good health. Based on the epidemiologic evidence, there is no reason to think that such a healthy eating pattern could not include eggs."

Combine the present belief that eggs do not contribute to the risk of heart disease with new scientific findings that eggs are lower in cholesterol than originally believed and you have a green light to enjoy a delicious breakfast featuring eggs. According to recently updated United States Department of Agriculture (USDA) nutrition data, eggs are lower in cholesterol than previously recorded. The USDA reports the nutrient composition of standard large eggs shows the average amount of cholesterol in one large egg is 185mg, down from 215mg, a 14 percent decrease. The analysis also revealed that one large egg provides nearly 11% daily value of vitamin D.

The American Heart Association now concedes that healthy adults can enjoy an egg a day without increasing their risk for heart disease, particularly if individuals opt for low cholesterol foods in the overall diet. This is good news for bariatric patients who are watching their cholesterol while following a high protein diet because whole eggs, including the long-avoided yolk, are a prime source of quality protein

INSIDE THE SHELL: EGG NUTRIENTS

For only 70 calories each, eggs are rich in nutrients. They contain, in varying amounts, almost every essential vitamin and mineral needed by humans. Egg protein is the standard by which other protein sources are measured. A large egg contains over six grams of protein, 4.5 grams of fat (1.5 saturated), and less than 1-gram carbohydrate.

According the American Egg Board (AEB) independent scientific findings conclude eggs are a stellar source of high-quality protein that sustains energy throughout the day and supports weight management goals. From the AEB media release titled, High-quality Protein at Breakfast and Weight Management:

"Eggs are all-natural and provide one of the highest quality proteins of any food available. One egg provides more than six grams of protein, or 13 percent of the recommended Daily Value (DV), and nearly half is found in the yolk. In fact, the protein quality in an egg is so high that the scientists often use eggs as the standard for measuring the protein quality of other foods.

"The all-natural, high-quality protein, like the protein in eggs, helps build muscles and allows you to feel full longer and stay energized, which can help you maintain a healthy weight. In fact, eating eggs for breakfast reduces hunger and decreases calorie consumption at lunch and throughout the day. The protein in eggs provides steady and sustained energy because it does not cause a surge in blood sugar or insulin levels, which can lead to a rebound effect or energy "crash" as blood sugar levels drop. In addition to providing nutrient-rich high-quality protein, eggs provide varying amounts of several B vitamins required to produce energy in the body, such as thiamin, riboflavin, folate, B12 and B6. And not only does the protein in eggs help kids and active adults build muscle strength, high-quality protein may help older adults prevent age-related muscle loss.

"Dietary protein intake directly influences muscle mass, strength and function in people of all ages. The six grams of high-quality protein in eggs can help active individuals build and preserve muscle, and help adults prevent muscle loss. Consuming protein foods, like eggs, following exercise can maximize muscle repair."

EGG BUYING CHECKLIST

While other food costs have skyrocketed, eggs continue to be one of nature's best bargains among high-quality protein foods. In 2014 eggs averaged less than $2 a dozen and they can often be found on sale for less.

An egg carton is marked with detailed information about the eggs it contains and once the cryptic markings are understood we have the knowledge to buy the best fresh quality eggs available. Here are a few things to look for when purchasing your next dozen eggs:

USDA Shield: The official USDA grade shield certifies the eggs were packaged and certified under federal supervision and the grades and weight classes were assigned by the USDA. It also indicates the production plant has been inspected for sanitation and operating procedures. A variety of images represent the USDA Shield. Look for a symbol (a shield shape or circle are most common) bearing the acronym "USDA" and may also include the words "Grade A" or "Inspected" or "Certified".

Expiration/Best By Date: On USDA grade-shielded egg cartons if an expiration date appears it can be no more than 30 days after the pack date. If a "Best by" or "Use by" date appears it can be no more than 45 days after the pack date. Remember, eggs kept in their carton and stored in the refrigerator at 45-degrees Fahrenheit are safe for use up to five weeks after purchase without a loss of quality. Currently the FDA advises storing eggs in the purchase carton rather than the refrigerator's built-in egg-keeping compartments or door shelving.

> ✳ *Hint:* Keeping eggs in their purchase carton is an effective way to monitor freshness and ensure they are used before their expiration date.

Know the Grade: Eggs available to consumers are graded AA, A, and B. The grade is assessed on the appearance of the egg when broken out, not the size or nutritive quality of the egg. Consumers generally only see grades AA and A on the store shelf; B grade eggs go to institutional egg users such as bakeries or food service operations. The USDA defines egg grade thusly:

Grade AA: Egg content covers a small area. White is firm, has much thick white surrounding the yolk and a small amount of thin white. The yolk is round and upstanding. Grade AA and Grade A eggs are best for frying and poaching where appearance is important.

Grade A: Egg content covers a moderate area. White is reasonably firm and has a considerable amount of thick white and a medium amount of thin white. The yolk is round and upstanding. This is the quality most often sold in stores.

Grade B: Egg content covers a very wide area. The yolk is enlarged and flattened.

Size Matters: Size tells you the minimum required net weight per dozen eggs. It does not refer to the dimensions of an egg or how big it looks. While some eggs in the carton may look slightly larger or smaller than the rest, it is the total weight of the dozen eggs that puts them in one of the following classes:

Jumbo: 30 ounces net weight per dozen or greater than 2.5 ounces per egg

Extra Large: 27 ounces net weight per dozen or greater than 2.25 ounces per egg

Large: 24 ounces net weight per dozen or greater than 2 ounces per egg

Medium: 21 ounces net weight per dozen or greater than 1.75 ounces per egg

Small: 18 ounces net weight per dozen or greater than 1.5 ounces per egg

Recipe Rule: For continuity most recipes published in the US are developed and tested using large 2-ounce eggs, the most common size of chicken egg available. In this LivingAfterWLS Publication all recipes have been triple-tested and recipes calling for eggs are always tested with large Grade AA or Grade A commercially produced "Large" chicken eggs. Nutritional information is calculated based on the standard use of large size eggs.

Shell Color: The eggshell color has no relationship to egg quality, flavor, nutritive value, cooking characteristics or shell thickness. An egg's shell color is determined by the breed of hen laying the egg. Brown eggs can be more costly than white eggs because brown-egg layers are larger birds and more costly to nurture for egg production than the smaller chickens laying white eggs. Brown eggs are preferred in New England while the rest of the country typically consumes white shell eggs.

Safe Purchase and Handling

Beyond looking at carton markings take the following measures to buy and keep eggs safe: buy eggs only if sold from a refrigerator or refrigerated case; open the carton and make sure that the eggs are clean and the shells are not cracked; refrigerate promptly; store eggs in their original carton and use them before the "Best by" date.

Farm Stand and Farmer's Market Eggs: While the FDA regulates the safe food production of commercial egg growers it is up the agriculture department in each US state and territory to regulate the safety of eggs produced at small farm operations for direct selling to customers at farm stands and farmer's markets. Within the states county health agencies are tasked with ensuring the safety of foods sold at small vendor markets. Check for regulations in your area by visiting your county extension service or visiting your state's department of agriculture website.

Fast and Easy Eggs

Now that we have a comprehensive understanding of the nutritional benefits of eggs and purchasing guidelines it is time to enjoy the health benefits of this so-called perfect protein. Eggs are an outstanding menu option any time of day but for our purposes in this Breakfast Basics publication we focus on two cooking methods that will get the day off to a good protein powered start: hard-cooked eggs and microwave cooked eggs. Each method includes a variety of ingredients to suit different tastes and the preparation and clean-up is efficient: all recipes can be completed in 15 minutes or less. Additionally, these recipes can be adjusted and tweaked to personal preference providing variety that helps avoid gastronomic boredom.

Hard Cooked Eggs

"Research shows that eating high-quality protein foods for breakfast, like eggs, can help you feel more satisfied and energized throughout the day. Make a batch of hard-boiled eggs so you'll have an all-natural, high-quality protein on-the-go meal or snack ready for the busy week ahead." American Egg Board. Visit http://www.incredibleegg.org

Method: Hard Cooked Eggs As instructed by the American Egg Board: Place as many eggs as desired in a single layer in a saucepan. Add enough water to come at least 1 inch above the eggs. Cover saucepan and place on high heat and bring water to a boil. As soon as the water begins to boil turn off heat and remove saucepan from stove. Keep the saucepan covered and let eggs sit in the hot water for 12 to 15-minutes. When time is up run cold water over eggs to cool them. To remove shell, crackle it by tapping gently all over. Roll egg between hands to loosen shell. Peel the eggs starting at the large end. Hold egg under running cold water or dip in bowl of water to help ease off shell. Once they are cooled store hard cooked eggs (in the shell) in the refrigerator, separated from raw eggs, and use within one week of cooking.

Note: Sometimes hard cooked eggs are card "hard boiled eggs". The food industry in recent years has shied away from this description in favor of hard cooked eggs to better describe the approved cooking method described above. Shell eggs that are overcooked in boiling water tend to be rubbery and unpleasant. The above cooking method produces a firm yet tender egg white and firm yet moist egg yolk that is safe to eat and pleasing to the palate.

Egg Cookers: At our house we prepare hard cooked eggs in an electric egg cooker, a small countertop appliance that uses steam to cook the eggs. The process is straightforward, takes under 10 minutes, and requires no tending. Egg cookers can be found with small kitchen appliances and can cost from $20 to $60 depending upon brand and options.

Hard Cooked Egg Possibilities

Following the directions above prepare 6 to 12 hard cooked eggs for convenient use throughout the week. Consider these serving possibilities and remember each hard-cooked egg provides about six grams of protein along with health promoting nutrients and minerals. While I firmly believe in abiding the "No Snacking" rule of weight loss surgery there are times when after a fair assessment of all considerations that I need a snack. If I wisely select a hard-cooked egg on its own in one of the following preparations I do not catapult my diet into chaos and non-compliance. An egg snack is perhaps the smartest way I know to break the "No Snacking" rule. Keeping hard cooked eggs available eliminates the hesitation I might feel were they not within reach when the need arises. It goes with the known diet hazard that we eat what is at hand; for me it makes sense to ensure this convenient and smart snack is suitably available.

Chilled Egg Plates:

These breakfast meals take advantage of chilled hard cooked eggs, meat, and cheese for the protein source and benefit from the addition of seasonal fruit, berries, and vegetables for a nutritional start to the morning. Consider packing your ingredients in a sectioned container *(sometimes called a Bento Box)* the night before and enjoy your chilled egg plate as part of your morning routine.

CITRUS SUNRISE

Arrange two hard cooked, peeled and quartered eggs on a plate with sliced meat (leftover turkey, chicken, or roast beef are good choices), sliced cheese, and orange segments.

CAPRESE LAYERS

Arrange sliced tomatoes, sliced mozzarella, and sliced hard cooked eggs on a plate. Drizzle with vinaigrette and garnish with chopped fresh basil for a delightful breakfast salad.

SHRIMP COCKTAIL

Mix 1 finely chopped hard cooked egg with 1/4-cup prepared cocktail sauce, and a squeeze of fresh lemon. Arrange 6 to 8 ready-to-eat peeled and deveined shrimp on a plate with one hard cooked, peeled and quartered egg, and serve with cocktail sauce. Garnish with lemon wedge. Shrimp provide 6 grams of protein per ounce, are low in calories, and rich in nutrients including the B vitamins and antioxidants.

APPLE FOLLY

Wash and core a large tart green apple, cut into 1/4-inch slices and arrange on a plate. In a small bowl mix 1/3-cup olive oil mayonnaise with 1/4-teaspoon ground cinnamon and spread apple slices with cinnamon mayonnaise. Slice two hard cooked eggs; top each apple slice

That's a Wrap

Use medium-thickness sliced low-sodium deli meat as a "wrap" for the spread to increase protein values and provide variety. To make wraps (also called rolls or pinwheels) spread 1-2 tablespoons egg spread along the long edge of a meat slice and roll tightly, wrap with plastic wrap or waxed paper and refrigerate 2 hours before slicing. Try using a thin layer of cream cheese on the meat before adding the egg spread to help "glue" the wrap when rolled. Serve meat wraps with dill pickle slices.

Green Eggs

Add 1/2 mashed avocado (about 1/2-cup) to the original recipe for smooth flavor and beneficial monounsaturated fat. A squeeze of fresh lemon or lime will prevent the avocado from browning due to oxidation.

Some Like it Hot

Turn up the heat with a shake or two of tabasco sauce or your favorite hot sauce. Mixtures that contain fish or red meat benefit from the addition of prepared horseradish sauce.

* *Hint:* Consider using plain unflavored yogurt in place of mayonnaise or dressing as the binding ingredient in any hard-cooked egg preparation. Yogurt provides the texture of a more traditional binding ingredient in addition to the nutrients and protein which are absent other ingredients which tend to be higher in fat.

Warm Hard Cooked Egg Meals

These clever breakfast dishes take advantage of prepared ingredients, including hard cooked eggs, which are assembled and warmed immediately before serving. Prepare and refrigerate hard cooked eggs, then warm as directed in the recipe preparation directions.

English Muffin Egg Pizzas

Toast one whole grain English muffin half. Layer with 1 tablespoon jarred spaghetti sauce, one sliced hard cooked egg, and 1 tablespoon shredded cheese. Microwave 30 seconds on high or until cheese melts. Add 1 ounce chopped Canadian bacon if desired.

California Melt

Toast one whole grain English muffin half. Spread with 1 tablespoon cream cheese, top with 1 slice fresh tomato, 1 hard cooked egg, sliced: and 2-3 slices fresh avocado. Microwave 30 seconds on high until warm. Add a dash of sriracha sauce for exciting flavor.

Fiesta Quesadilla

Mix 2 coarsely chopped hard cooked eggs with 2 ounces shredded cheese and 1/4 cup prepared salsa. Place mixture on one half whole grain tortilla, fold over. Heat non-stick skillet over medium heat and cook quesadilla, turning once, until cheese melts and tortilla is lightly browned. Alternatively, wrap quesadilla in waxed or parchment paper and heat 30 to 60 seconds in microwave oven until cheese melts and quesadilla is warm. Serve with additional salsa and sour cream or plain non-fat yogurt.

Turkey Sausage Melts

This preparation takes advantage of ready-to-serve fully cooked sausage. We tested the recipe with Jimmy Dean® Fully Cooked Turkey Sausage Patties that can be found in the refrigerated meats section at your supermarket. They are packaged 2 patties per pouch and a serving of 2 patties provides 100 calories, 11 grams protein, 7 grams fat, 1-gram carbohydrate. To prepare microwave sausage follow manufacturer's instructions. Top each heated sausage patties with 1 sliced hard cooked egg and 1 slice Cheddar cheese. Microwave an additional 30 seconds or until cheese melts: serve immediately.

Fast Food: Eggs in 5 Minutes or Less

Have you discovered the wonderful world of microwave cooked eggs? For years I was intimidated by cooking eggs, and between you and me, I was horribly unsuccessful at cooking eggs. There is a skillet with burnt-on eggs hidden in the "back forty" to prove it! But don't despair, the microwave cooking method changed my life and it can do the same for you!

Once you get this method down unleash your inner gourmet, peruse your refrigerator for ingredients, and serve a meal in a mug every day. Remember to always coat the mug or bowl with cooking spray to prevent the food from sticking. Skipping this step will result in a dishwashing nightmare (yes! That's experience talking.) It may take a few attempts to learn how long it takes to cook eggs in your microwave oven, don't be afraid to experiment, always starting with the lowest cooking time (usually about 30 seconds) and adding more time as necessary, usually 10-15 seconds at a time. Until you are familiar with how your microwave oven cooks eggs never exceed 30 seconds per interval to avoid overcooking and burning the eggs.

Use caution to avoid over cooking or under cooking. And remember, eggs will continue to cook and firm up after removed from microwave, so allow them to set and cool a couple of minutes before enjoying.

If you want to microwave eggs for an omelet or wrap use a shallow dinner plate with a higher rim for cooking; use a small mixing bowl to beat eggs, pour onto plate sprayed with cooking spray. A soup bowl will work well for cooking three to four eggs at once. Ramekins or custard dishes also work well, usually for cooking a single egg.

Caution: It's Hot! Always use an oven mitt or hot pad when removing your egg mug or bowl from the microwave oven: it will be hot. It may be handy to use a plate or saucer to set the hot cooking vessel on when serving.

Warning! Never attempt to "hard boil" an egg in the shell in the microwave, unless of course you can dispose of the microwave oven out on the back forty. Huge Mess! The American Egg Board says, "Never microwave eggs in shells. Steam builds up too quickly inside the egg therefore eggs are likely to explode."

Food Safety Note: Do not use the same fork to stir the raw eggs that you use to eat the cooked eggs. Put the cooking fork in the dishwasher and use a clean fork for eating to avoid the potential for food borne illness caused by cross contamination.

BASIC MICROWAVE COFFEE CUP SCRAMBLE

Try this recipe first. It is the basic cooking method that is used for all of the microwave scrambles and breakfast bowls.

Ingredients:
2 eggs
2 tablespoons milk
2 tablespoons shredded cheese
salt and pepper for seasoning

Coat a 12-ounce microwave-safe coffee mug or bowl with cooking spray. Add eggs and milk; beat with a fork until blended. Microwave on high 30 seconds; remove and stir. Microwave 30 seconds, check for doneness, microwave additional time at 10-second increments until egg is set. Use a hot pad to remove from microwave; allow to rest 1-2 minutes. Top with cheese and season with salt and pepper. This two-egg serving provides 215 calories; 17 grams protein; 15 grams fat (6 grams saturated); 2 grams carbohydrate.

1-Minute Ham and Egg Breakfast

Eggs, ham and cheese join forces in a three-ingredient hot breakfast providing hunger satisfying protein prepared fast and mess-free. This is a good use of left-over ham, chicken, or turkey.

Ingredients:
1 or 2 eggs
1-ounce ham, chopped
1 tablespoon shredded cheese

Directions: Coat a 12-ounce microwave-safe coffee mug or bowl with cooking spray. Add eggs and beat with a fork until blended. Microwave on high 30 seconds; remove and stir. Top with chopped ham and shredded cheese; microwave 30 seconds, check for doneness; microwave additional time at 10-second increments until egg is set. Allow to rest 1-2 minutes. Season with salt and pepper and enjoy.

Using 1 egg this recipe serves one and provides 133 calories; 12 grams protein; 8 grams fat (3 saturated); 2 grams carbohydrate. With 2 eggs provides 205 calories; 18 grams protein; 12 grams fat (4.5 saturated); and 2.5 grams carbohydrate.

VEGGIE EGG SCRAMBLE

Use vegetables from last night's dinner reinvented in this scrambled egg morning meal. Cooked vegetables such as sautéed greens, mushrooms, broccoli, bell peppers, and asparagus are especially tasty. Use fresh tomato slices for a garnish and your day begins with a smile!

Ingredients:
1 or 2 eggs
1 tablespoon water
1/4 cup cooked vegetables of your choice
1 tablespoon shredded cheese
fresh tomatoes, sliced (optional)

Directions: Coat a 12-ounce microwave-safe coffee mug or bowl with cooking spray. Add eggs and water; beat with a fork until blended. Microwave on high 30 seconds; remove and stir. Fold the vegetables into eggs, top with shredded cheese. Microwave 30 seconds, check for doneness; microwave additional time at 10-second increments until egg is set. Allow to rest and cool 1-2 minutes. Garnish with fresh tomato, season with salt and pepper and enjoy immediately.

Using 1 egg this recipe serves one and provides approximately 110 calories; 10 grams protein; 6 grams fat (2 saturated); 3 grams carbohydrate. With 2 eggs recipe provides 188 calories; 17 grams protein; 12 grams fat (4.5 saturated); and 4.5 grams carbohydrate.

Egg, Sausage & Tomato Breakfast Bowl

If this turns out to be one of your favorites, try this: cook a package of bulk breakfast sausage (also called rolled sausage) when preparing your meals for the week. Break sausage into crumbles, like ground cooked taco meat. Store in an air-tight container from which you can quickly take the needed amount as you prepare your breakfast bowl.

Ingredients:
2 eggs
2 tablespoons milk
2 tablespoons fully cooked breakfast sausage crumbles or 1 fully cooked breakfast sausage link or patty, chopped
1 tablespoon finely shredded Cheddar cheese
2 tablespoons chopped tomato
2 basil leaves, thinly sliced (delightful, but optional)

Directions: Coat a microwave-safe soup bowl with cooking spray. Add eggs and milk and beat with a fork until blended, fold in sausage. Microwave on high 30 seconds; remove and stir. Top with shredded cheese and chopped tomato. Microwave 30 seconds, check for doneness; microwave additional time at 10-to-15-second increments until egg is set. Garnish with fresh basil, season with salt and pepper and enjoy immediately. Serves one providing about 230 calories; 19 grams protein; 16 grams fat (6 saturated); and 4 grams carbohydrate.

Salsa in the Morning Mug Scramble

No need to wait in the drive through for a Mexican breakfast to go: this recipe is ready before you can say 'ole! Take it up a notch using last night's left-over taco ingredients including seasoned cooked ground meat, beans, and top with sour cream, guacamole, salsa, and cheese.

Ingredients:
2 eggs
1 teaspoon butter or spread*
2 tablespoons prepared salsa
2 tablespoons shredded Mexican cheese blend
Salsa, sour cream or guacamole, if desired

Directions: Coat a microwave-safe soup bowl with cooking spray. Add eggs and butter or spread and beat with a fork until blended. Microwave on high 30 seconds; remove and stir. Fold in salsa, top with shredded cheese; microwave 30 seconds, check for doneness, microwave additional time at 10-second increments until egg is set. Serve with additional salsa, sour cream, and guacamole, as desired. Serves one providing about 230 calories; 13 grams protein; 10 grams fat (4 saturated); and 18 grams carbohydrate.

*As an alternative to butter try using a spread made with yogurt such as Brummel & Brown (the one in the blue tub sold by the butter and margarine in the refrigerator case). This spread provides the sweet creamy taste of butter and the wholesome health benefits of yogurt with 1/4 the calories of butter and no trans-fat.

Muggy Eggs Breakfast Bar

I'm using the term "breakfast bar" loosely to describe the advance preparation of ingredients to make the creation of a morning egg mug a breeze. Consider gathering any of the ingredients listed –or anything you enjoy – to keep on hand in the refrigerator. Organize breakfast bar ingredients in easy-to-access containers or resealable plastic bags and store in one location for easy access. With a few select items and a dozen eggs you can have a warm protein first meal to start the day, even on the most hectic mornings. Simply use a few supplies and the basic method for cooking microwave mug eggs and build your original breakfast creation one scrumptious mug at a time. For example, chop left-over fried chicken, add to eggs, top with ready-to-eat country gravy and enjoy a breakfast so yummy you'll be happy all day long!

Here are some suggested ingredients to get you started:

Animal Protein: Cooked ground meat; cooked steak or pork chops, sliced; cooked shredded poultry; chopped Canadian bacon; cooked sausage, crumbled and drained; bacon, cooked drained of fat and crumbled; canned fish; cooked fish fillets, flaked; deli meat, sliced and chopped; seafood including shrimp, scallops, lobster, etc., cooked and chopped.

Dairy: Eggs, cottage cheese; sour cream; assorted varieties shredded cheese; milk; butter; pasteurized egg product (Egg Beaters®).

Vegetables: Any cooked vegetables including asparagus; bell peppers; broccoli; carrots; cooked greens (chard, spinach, kale); sautéed celery or fennel; legumes including canned beans and canned refried beans; mushrooms; onions or leeks; snow peas; green and yellow snap beans; tomatoes both raw and cooked (canned); summer squash (zucchini, crookneck; cooked and mashed winter squash (acorn, banana, butternut, pumpkin, and spaghetti squash).

Condiments: Salsa, green chili sauce, spaghetti, marinara, and alfredo sauce, tapenade, bruschetta-style tomato sauce, pesto, hummus, mayonnaise, mustard, ketchup, gravy (ready-to-serve), assorted vinaigrettes and salad dressings.

Helpful Hints and Tips

- Double-check the mug or bowl intended for cooking your eggs to ensure it is safe for microwave cooking. Use hot pads to handle mugs and bowls which become quite hot during cooking.
- Always use cooking spray to liberally coat the inside of the mug or bowl before microwave cooking eggs. Try olive oil or butter flavored sprays. Cooking spray is the best ingredient to use to prevent stuck-on eggs that make clean-up nearly impossible.
- If you enjoy sautéed vegetables in your eggs cook a batch on the weekend; store refrigerated in a tightly covered container; add by the spoonful to your mug egg concoction during the week. (I like a mixture of chopped onion, celery, bell pepper, and mushrooms.) Leftover vegetables can also serve this purpose.
- Fresh fruit or berries are a sweet and flavorful side dish compliment to the Basic Microwave Coffee Cup Scramble. Including a few bites of melon, strawberries, grapes and other fresh fruits and berries is a smart strategy for preempting sugar cravings later in the morning.
- For a boost of energy in the afternoon make a coffee mug scramble. The protein will satisfy hunger cravings and provide an energy boost without the negative "carb-coma" effect of a non-nutritional simple carbohydrate snack.

Eggs are inexpensive. Practice. Experiment. Enjoy!

Make-Ahead Breakfast Burrito

When you have extra taco fixings try this make-ahead breakfast: Prepare the mug scramble with the desired taco ingredients, cool, roll burrito-style in a 6-inch tortilla and wrap securely in plastic cling wrap. Refrigerate overnight and simply reheat in the microwave oven. This works best with the warm taco ingredients: lettuce and salad-type ingredients are not recommended for including in the egg burrito. However, they are a nice "side dish" compliment to the burrito if time allows. We enjoy this handy breakfast so much that I intentionally prepare extra taco ingredients for this purpose. Bonus: cook and clean one meal for the price of two!

Mama Mia Egg Lasagna

This recipe is a shake more complicated than the basic mug eggs. But it is certainly worth the effort when time allows and is delightful served for a brunch buffet.

Ingredients:
4 eggs
1 teaspoon Italian herb seasoning blend
2 tablespoons milk or evaporated milk
1/4 cup cottage cheese or ricotta cheese
1/4 cup tablespoons prepared marinara sauce
2 tablespoons shredded mozzarella cheese
Parmesan cheese for garnish.

Directions: in a medium mixing bowl sprayed with cooking spray add eggs, Italian seasoning blend, and milk; beat until smooth. Microwave on high 75 seconds; remove and stir; cook an additional 30 seconds or until soft curds form but eggs are still wet. Spray two 12-

ounce microwave safe mugs with cooking spray. Place 1/4 of egg mixture in each mug, layer with 1 tablespoon ricotta and 1 tablespoon marinara sauce; repeat layers finishing with sauce. Top each mug with half of the shredded mozzarella and microwave separately 30 seconds or until eggs are set. Allow to rest before garnishing with Parmesan cheese. Season with salt and pepper and enjoy

Hot Skillet Meals

At our house a hot skillet breakfast is a luxury most enjoyed during winter weekends when we are homebound, and life is moving at a slower pace. How about at your house? Hopefully we can all find time for a warm morning meal occasionally. With mindfully selected ingredients skillet meals can be quite high in protein and made more flavorful with the addition of vegetables, fruit, and cheese. Let's get that frying pan heated and get the skillet party started!

Glossary: Traditional Breakfast Meats

Bacon is a type of salt-cured pork. Bacon is prepared from several different cuts of meat, typically from the pork belly or from back cuts, which have less fat than the belly. It is eaten on its own, as a side dish, or used as a minor ingredient to flavor dishes. Nutrition: 1 slice (standard thickness) provides 44 calories, 3 grams protein, 3.5 grams fat, 0 carbohydrates. Check package label for sodium and potassium values.

Ham is pork from a leg cut that has been preserved by wet or dry curing, with or without smoking. Ham is produced from whole cuts of meat as well as meat cuts that are mechanically formed to a desirable shape, such as sandwich cuts. Sodium is used in curing and seasoning which results in a high sodium value per servings, sometimes as high as 40% of the daily value. Check labels to find a ham product suited to your needs. *Nutrition:* 3-ounce serving is 125 calories, 18 grams protein, 5 grams fat, and 1 gram carbohydrate.

Canadian Bacon also known as "back bacon" is made only from the lean eye of the pork loin. It is smoked, trimmed into cylindrical medallions, and thickly sliced. It is packaged fully cooked and ready to eat. *Nutrition:* 2 (1-ounce) slices: 90 calories, 12 grams protein, 4-grams fat, 1-gram carbohydrate. Check package label for sodium and potassium values.

Sausage and Sausages refers to a meat product usually made from ground meat, often pork, beef, or poultry. Seasoning including salt, spices and sometimes regional flavorings including herbs. Sausage can refer to the loose sausage meat which is called bulk sausage and means the sausage is not enclosed in casing. Sausages, the plural form, generally describes the meat mixture encased in a tubular skin or casing. In the recipes presented here we use bulk sausage or fresh sausages.

Bulk Sausage, or sometimes sausage meat or skinless sausage, refers to raw, ground, spiced meat, usually sold without any casing.

Fresh Sausages are made from uncured meats in casing. They can be finger sized or larger. Fresh sausages must be thoroughly cooked before eating. Some brands call this product "breakfast sausage".

SCRAMBLED EGGS

When the schedule permits nothing beats a freshly prepared warm egg breakfast enjoyed as a meal at the table. A few select ingredients added to nutritional and economical eggs turn breakfast into a meal to savor. These recipes make 2-6 servings providing for guests at your table or go-to leftovers sure to satisfy hunger cravings.

BASIC SCRAMBLED EGGS

Follow this recipe for basic scrambled eggs. Look to the suggested additions for delicious and exciting ways to take your breakfast scramble to the next level.

Ingredients:
6 eggs
1 teaspoon salt
3 tablespoons water
1 tablespoon canola oil

Directions: Heat oil in a medium non-stick 10-inch skillet over medium heat. Meanwhile in a medium bowl beat eggs, salt and water with a fork or whisk until well blended. Pour eggs into skillet and watch closely. As eggs begin to set at the bottom and side, gently lift cooked portions with spatula so that thin, uncooked portion can flow to bottom. Avoid constant stirring as this toughens the proteins making the egg texture rubbery. Cook 3 to 5 minutes until eggs are thickened and set but still moist. Serve warm. Season with salt and pepper. Serves 4. One serving provides 180 calories, 10 grams protein, 2 grams fat, zero carbohydrate.

CHILE CHEESE SCRAMBLE

Following the Basic Scrambled Eggs recipe add to the beaten eggs add 1 (4-ounce) can chopped green chiles, drained. Cook eggs as directed. Top with 1/2 cup shredded Cheddar cheese and 1 medium tomato diced. Serve warm. Season with salt and pepper.

Homestyle Scramble

Using the Basic Scrambled Eggs recipe heat the oil in a medium non-stick 10-inch skillet over medium heat. Add 1 cup refrigerated diced potatoes with onions, 1 ~~small zucchini~~, chopped, and 1 medium tomato chopped. Cook and stir until hot, about 6 minutes. Pour egg mixture over vegetable mixture and proceed to cook as directed in basic recipe. Season with salt and pepper.

Denver Scramble

Before adding eggs to pan cook 1/2 cup chopped fully cooked ham with 1/2 green bell pepper seeded and chopped and 1/2 medium onion diced in the oil, about 2 minutes. Spread ham and vegetables evenly on the bottom of the skillet, pour egg mixture over ham and vegetable mixture and proceed to cook as directed in basic recipe. Remove skillet from heat, sprinkle 1/2 cup shredded Swiss cheese on top of eggs, cover and let stand 5 minutes for cheese to melt and eggs to set. Serve warm. Season with salt and pepper.

California Scramble

Prepare eggs as directed in Basic Scrambled Eggs mixture, set aside. Dice 1 small avocado and 1 medium ripe tomato: set aside. In the skillet with oil cook 4 slices chopped bacon until crisp, remove from skillet and drain on paper towel. Wipe skillet clean, add 1 tablespoon of oil and heat, add the eggs and proceed to cook as directed in basic recipe. When eggs are nearly done add cooked bacon and stir. Serve scrambled eggs topped with chopped avocado, chopped ripe tomato, and shredded Cheddar cheese. Season with salt and pepper.

Huevos Rancheros Scramble

Prepare eggs as directed in Basic Scrambled Eggs mixture adding 1/2 cup chunky-style salsa, set aside. heat the oil in a medium non-stick 10-inch skillet over medium heat. Add 1/2-pound uncooked chorizo or pork sausage and cook, stirring occasionally, until no longer pink. Remove from skillet, drain and set aside. Wipe skillet clean, add 1 tablespoon of oil and heat, add the eggs and proceed to cook as directed in basic recipe. When eggs are nearly done add cooked chorizo or sausage and stir. Serve scrambled eggs with additional salsa and shredded Cheddar cheese.

Breakfast Tacos

This fun take on traditional meat and bean tacos is at equally at home on the breakfast and supper plate. Vary the toppings offered to suit your taste.

Ingredients:
8 eggs
Salt and pepper
1 tablespoon canola oil
1 medium red bell pepper, chopped
1 medium yellow onion, chopped
1 (8-ounce) package shredded pepper Jack cheese
6 ready-to-eat corn taco shells
1 cup shredded lettuce
1 small avocado, pitted, peeled and sliced
1 medium ripe tomato, diced
Toppings: chunky-style salsa, sour cream, taco sauce, chopped green onion, sliced black olives, black beans, rinsed and drained.

Directions: In a medium bowl beat eggs, season with salt and pepper, set aside. Heat oil in a medium non-stick 10-inch skillet over medium heat. Add bell pepper and onion and cook and stir until tender, about 5 minutes. Pour eggs into skillet with vegetables and watch closely. As eggs begin to set at the bottom and side, gently lift cooked portions with spatula so that thin, uncooked portion can flow to bottom. Cook 3 to 5 minutes until eggs are thickened and set but still moist. Gently stir in cheese. Remove eggs from heat. Heat taco shells as directed on package. Fill taco shells with lettuce, 1/6-portion of the eggs, avocado, and tomato. Add toppings as desired. Serve warm.

Scrambled Eggs on Caramelized Onions

This is a complete meal that is appropriate for breakfast, lunch, or dinner. Enjoy the eggs with a side serving of fresh fruit and berries.

Ingredients:
4 tablespoons unsalted butter
2 medium-sized yellow onions, sliced very thin
salt and freshly ground pepper
4 to 6 eggs, beaten
3 tablespoons water
Chopped chives, chervil or parsley for garnish (optional)

Directions: Melt 2 tablespoons of butter in a heavy skillet set over medium heat. Reduce the heat to low and add the onions. Cover the pan and cook until the onions are very soft and caramel-colored about 10 minutes. Season with salt and pepper and set aside. Beat the eggs and water together, adding a pinch of salt and pepper. Melt the remaining 2 tablespoons butter in a small skillet (preferably non-stick) over medium heat. Pour in the beaten eggs and add salt and pepper to taste. Scramble to desired doneness. Divide the onions between two dinner plates, creating a bed of caramelized onions. Spoon eggs on top and garnish if desired with fresh herbs. Serve immediately. Makes 2 servings.

Spicy Shakshuka

The New York Times calls Shakshuka "the apex of eggs-for-dinner recipes, though in Israel it is breakfast food, a bright, spicy start to the day." This popular recipe originates in North Africa with countless regional variations to the basic formula. Most North American versions top the spicy sauce with cool smooth feta cheese which softens into creamy nuggets as the eggs bake. Make it for brunch, lunch or supper and enjoy often.

Ingredients
8 large eggs
3 Tbsp. olive oil
1 onion, chopped
1 red pepper, chopped
2 cloves garlic, minced
1 teaspoon each chili powder, ground cumin and paprika
Salt and pepper to taste
3 tablespoons tomato paste
1 (28-ounce) can San Marzano peeled tomatoes
1/3 cup feta cheese, finely crumbled
1/4 cup chopped fresh cilantro or parsley

Directions: Heat oven to 400°F. Heat oil in a large ovenproof skillet set over medium heat. Add onion, red pepper, garlic, chili powder, cumin, paprika, salt, pepper and cayenne and cook and stir for 5 minutes or until vegetables start to soften. Stir in tomato paste; continue cooking for 1 minute. Crush or mash San Marzano tomatoes, keeping juices. Add tomatoes to skillet; bring to simmer. Reduce heat to medium-low. Cook stirring occasionally, for about 15 minutes or until sauce has thickened.

Leaving sauce in the skillet make 8 indents in the sauce with spoon, crack egg into each indent. Transfer to oven. Cook for 5 to 8 minutes or until eggs are soft-cooked or until desired doneness. Garnish with feta cheese and cilantro. Each serving of 1 egg and 1/3 cup sauce with cheese provides 170 calories, 9 grams protein, 11 grams fat, 9 grams carbohydrate.

SEAFOOD SCRAMBLE

This is a delicious special occasion brunch-style entrée. You can substitute imitation seafood flakes if you prefer. The large batch is intended to serve six. Leftover portions may be refrigerated up to three days and gently reheated in the microwave before enjoying.

Ingredients:
1 (7-ounce) package frozen shrimp
1 (7-ounce) can King crab, flaked and drained
3 tablespoons sweet cream butter
2 tablespoons flour
3/4 cup half-and-half or milk
1 tablespoon green onion tops, chopped
1 tablespoon green onion bottoms, chopped
12 eggs
1 1/2 teaspoon salt
1/4 teaspoon black pepper
Tabasco, to taste
4 tablespoons butter
1/8 teaspoon seafood seasoning

Directions: Mix prepared seafood together and set aside. Blend butter and flour in large skillet. Cook until smooth. Slowly add half and half or milk. Cook until it starts to thicken, approximately 1 minute. Stir in onions and seafood. In second skillet melt 4 tablespoons of butter; add beaten eggs and spices. Gently cook eggs. As they begin to set, gradually add your seafood mixture. Cook until thick and creamy. Serves 6.

CONFETTI SCRAMBLE

Ingredients:
1 to 1 1/2 cups kernel corn (cut fresh from cobs, thawed frozen or drained canned)
1/4 cup chopped green pepper
2 tablespoons chopped sweet red pepper or pimiento
2 tablespoons chopped onion
1 teaspoon to 2 tablespoons butter or cooking oil OR cooking spray
8 eggs
1/2 cup skim or low-fat milk
1/2 teaspoon seasoned salt, optional
Green and/or sweet red pepper rings, optional

Directions: In 10-inch omelet pan or skillet over medium heat or hot coals, cook corn, peppers and onion in butter until tender but not brown, about 5 to 7 minutes. Meanwhile, in large bowl, beat together eggs and milk with salt, if desired, until blended. Pour over vegetables. As mixture begins to set, gently draw an inverted pancake turner completely across bottom and sides of pan, forming large soft curds. Continue until eggs are thickened and no visible liquid egg remains. Do not stir constantly. Garnish with pepper rings, if desired.

THE ONE-PAN BREAKFAST

I often here from men in our weight loss surgery community that they want a hearty, less fussy breakfast. A man breakfast if you will. Here is a blueprint for a manly one-pan breakfast. Use it as your guideline for tossing together great food in snap to start the day off right.

Ingredients:
6 strips bacon, cooked and crumbled
1 cup mushroom slices
1 cup grape tomatoes, washed, halved
Salt and Pepper to taste
Canola or olive oil
8 large eggs

Directions: Coat the bottom of a large skillet with the canola or olive oil, about 1 teaspoon. Heat over medium high and add the mushrooms and tomatoes. Cook and stir until vegetables are tender and lightly browned. Season with salt and pepper. Transfer mixture to a plate and keep warm. Add crumbled bacon to skillet and toss and stir until just reheated. Add warm crumbled bacon to mushroom and tomatoes. Add 2 teaspoons canola or olive oil to the pan and then carefully crack in the eggs. Cook them sunny side up, or until the whites are set but the yolks are still runny. As the eggs continue to cook distribute the bacon, mushrooms and tomatoes back to the pan arranging around the eggs. Cook eggs to your preferred doneness and serve warm, 2 eggs per serving, with a generous serving of the vegetables and bacon.

Changeups: Scramble the eggs if you prefer. When almost done top with bacon and veggies. Add a sprinkle of shredded cheese and melt under broiler. Consider using cooked flaked halibut or salmon in place of the bacon. Peeled, ready-to-eat shrimp is another good lean protein that works well in this dish. No time for veggies? Use good quality salsa in place of the vegetables.

Poached Eggs over Sautéed Spinach Greens

Well prepared poached eggs are a thing of beauty and the pride of many a chef. All it takes is a little practice to turn out beautiful perfectly cooked eggs. Poaching eggs is also a suitable method for cooking eggs to different levels of doneness from runny yolks to firm yolks and in between.

Ingredients:
4 eggs
1 tsp white wine vinegar
about 4 cups water
1 cup thinly sliced green onion
6 medium cloves garlic, sliced
4 cups fresh baby spinach
4 tablespoons chicken broth (divided)
juice & zest of one lemon
salt and black pepper to taste

Directions: Bring water and vinegar to a fast simmer in a skillet large enough to fit eggs. Make sure there is enough water to cover eggs. While water is coming to a simmer, heat 1 tablespoon broth in a separate stainless steel 10-inch skillet. Sauté sliced green onion in broth over medium heat for about 3 minutes. Add garlic slices and continue to sauté stirring constantly for another minute.

Add baby spinach, remaining broth, and lemon juice, and simmer covered on medium low heat for about 10 minutes stirring occasionally. Spinach will wilt down considerably. When done season by tossing with lemon zest, salt and pepper. Divide mixture among 4 plates.

In the boiling vinegar water poach eggs until desired doneness. This will take about 5 minutes, or just until the white is set and the yolk has filmed over. Remove from vinegar water with a slotted spoon and place on top of greens. One egg and 1/4 of the spinach mixture is a serving.

1¼ cup shredded Mexican cheese blend
3 medium green onions, sliced
1/3 cup baking mix
1 cup milk
4 eggs
Salt and pepper
1/4 cup chunky-style salsa
~~1/4 cup no-sugar-added peach preserves~~

Directions: Heat oven to 350°F. Spray a 9-inch glass pie plate with cooking spray. Evenly spread 1 cup shredded cheese and the sliced green onion in the pie plate. In a medium bowl whisk the baking mix, milk, and eggs until well blended, season with salt and pepper. Pour over cheese and onions and place in oven to bake 30 to 35 minutes. Test for doneness by inserting a knife in center. It will come out clean when the omelet is done. ~~In a small bowl combine the salsa and preserves~~, serve with salsa a wedge of baked omelet and garnish with remaining cheese. Serves 6. Each serving provides 230 calories, 12 grams protein, 8 grams fat, 17 grams carbohydrate.

<u>Bell Pepper and Vidalia Onion Strata with Fresh Salsa</u>

Provided by ChooseMyPlate, a service of the U.S. Department of Agriculture. ChooseMyPlate.gov

Loaded with sweet Vidalia onions and bell peppers, this delicious baked breakfast or brunch dish can be assembled ahead of time, leaving just the baking for the morning.

Ingredients
1 Vidalia onion, divided
1/2 red bell pepper, sliced vertically
1/2 green bell pepper, sliced vertically

1 tablespoon olive oil
4 large eggs
4 egg whites
1/2 cup skim milk
1/8 teaspoon ground black pepper
cooking spray
4 slices whole-grain bread toasted, cubed
1/2 cup reduced-fat Italian blend shredded cheese
10 cherry tomatoes or 2 tomatoes chopped
1 garlic clove, minced

Directions: Place rack in center of oven and preheat oven to 350 ºF. Cut Vidalia onion into slices vertically; reserve about 1/4 of onion. Heat oil in a 10-inch non-stick skillet. Sauté onion and pepper slices for 5-8 minutes, until tender and just starting to brown. Remove from heat. Beat eggs, egg whites, milk, and pepper in large bowl, set aside. Spray 8' or 9' baking pan (square or round) with cooking spray. Arrange bread cubes in bottom of pan. Sprinkle with shredded cheese. Add sautéed vegetables and pour in egg mix. Bake uncovered for 45 minutes, until set. Egg dishes should be cooked to 160 ºF. While strata is baking, prepare salsa, by dicing and mixing cherry tomatoes, garlic, and remaining Vidalia onion. Serving Suggestions: 1/2 cup cantaloupe chunks.

Serves 4. Nutrition per serving: 240 calories, 19 grams protein, 9 grams fat, 21 grams carbohydrate (4 grams dietary fiber, 8 grams sugar).

Spring Eggs with Salmon and Asparagus

Extra time and attention is needed for the successful preparation of this egg entrée. But the results are well worth the effort.

Ingredients:
- 8 large whole eggs
- 1/4 teaspoon salt
- 1/8 teaspoon pepper
- 2 tablespoons milk, 2% low-fat
- 1/4 teaspoon baking powder
- 1 tablespoon butter, chilled and quartered
- 8 ounces asparagus spears, peeled and sliced
- 2 ounces Asiago Cheese, shredded
- 4 ounces smoked salmon, flaked
- 2 ounces parsley sprigs, coarsely chopped

Directions: Place the oven rack in the lower third of the oven: heat oven to 325F. Liberally coat a 2-quart oven safe casserole dish with unflavored cooking spray. (Alternatively, coat four 6-ounce custard cups with cooking spray and place on baking sheet lined with parchment paper for easy clean-up.) In a medium bowl whisk eggs, salt, pepper, whole milk, and baking powder until slightly frothy and well blended. Pour mixture into prepared casserole or custard cups and bake 6 minutes. Remove from oven, stir with a fork, return to oven and bake 4 minutes, removing and stirring again. If eggs are curdled and near done to desired consistency evenly top them with the butter pieces, asparagus spears, shredded Asiago Cheese, and flaked smoked salmon. Return to oven a bake 2-4 minutes keeping a close watch. Remove them immediately when they reach your desired consistency. Garnish with chopped parsley.

Alternative Method: Cooks that are confident in their stove top skills may prepare these eggs in a skillet following the usual best practice and method for skillet scrambled eggs.

Store leftovers in single-serve microwave safe containers. Gently reheat 30 to 60 seconds and enjoy another high protein meal.

Spring Eggs Serves 4. Each serving provides 257 Calories; 21 grams protein; 17 grams fat (7 saturated); 4 grams carbohydrate; 1-gram dietary fiber. A good source of vitamin C, vitamin A, B-Vitamins including folacin (folate).

Serving Ideas: Serve warm with fresh buttermilk cheddar biscuits or warm buttered toast. Provide additional shredded Asiago Cheese and chopped parsley for garnish. In the summer vine ripened sliced tomatoes compliment this meal and provided heart health nutrients and sunshine sweet flavor.

INGREDIENT NOTE: ASPARAGUS

Young thin asparagus is a luxurious spring delicacy. Look for it at the market beginning in February. Bunches should be bundled tightly enough to prevent breakage, but loose enough to avoid collaring the tender vegetable spears. Store refrigerated, the cut ends of the stalks in water, until use. When properly stored young asparagus will stay fresh four to five days.

Larger asparagus may be slightly woody with tough outer fibers. Remove the tough fibers with a vegetable or carrot peeler. This reveals the tender insides while removing the tough outer fibers that some people with gastric conditions find difficult to digest.

QUICK BAKES

Baking need not be an all-day affair. In fact, a well-considered recipe that leaves your hands and attention free while it cooks may be just the ticket for a busy morning. Here are a few of my favorite quick bake breakfast recipes.

CLOUD EGGS

Provided by Incredible Egg: https://www.incredibleegg.org

This is a fun family recipe: make a cloud for everyone! Add orange slices for sunshine on a cloudy plate. Rather than heat the oven give the baking task to your toaster oven which will produce results equal to the big oven.

Ingredients:
2 large eggs
1/4 tsp. salt
1/4 cup Gruyere cheese, grated

Directions: Preheat oven to 450°F. Line baking sheet with parchment paper. Separate egg whites and yolks. Place egg whites in large bowl and yolks in small bowl. Season egg whites with salt. Using a whisk or electric mixer, beat egg whites until stiff peaks form. Gently fold in grated cheese. Spoon egg whites into 2 mounds on prepared baking sheet. Create a small dent in center of mound with back of a spoon. Bake for about 3 minutes or slightly golden. Remove from oven and place egg yolk gently in center of each egg white cloud. SEASON with salt. Bake for about 3 minutes or until yolks are just set to preferred firmness. Serves 2, 1 cloud per serving. Nutrition: 126 calories, 10 grams protein, 9 grams fat, 0 carbohydrates.

MAKE AHEAD BREAKFAST BISCUIT QUICHES

Provided by Incredible Egg: https://www.incredibleegg.org

Ingredients:

2/3 cup shredded Swiss cheese
1/3 cup finely chopped ham
1/4 cup finely chopped green onions
3 eggs
2 Tablespoons milk
Salt and pepper to taste
1 (12-ounce) package refrigerated buttermilk biscuits

Heat oven to 350°F. Combine cheese, ham and green onions in small bowl; mix well. Beat eggs, milk, salt and pepper in medium bowl until blended. Separate biscuits: press or roll each into a 5-inch round on lightly floured surface. Spray a standard size 12-cup muffin tin with cooking spray. Place 1 biscuit in each of 10 outer muffin cups, leaving the 2 cups in center of pan empty. Press biscuits firmly against bottom and sides of cups and form rim at top. Spoon 2 tablespoons cheese mixture into each cup. Pour in egg mixture, dividing evenly. Bake in center of 350°F oven until filling is set and biscuits are deep golden brown, 20 to 25 minutes. Cool slightly before removing from pan; serve warm. To prepare ahead cool and refrigerate until use. Reheat gently in microwave oven or warm in conventional oven for 10 minutes at 300°F. One muffin provides 168 calories, 7 grams protein, 8 grams fat, and 16 grams carbohydrate with no added sugar.

SURE TO PLEASE BAKED EGGS & CHEESE

Provided by ChooseMyPlate, a service of the U.S. Department of Agriculture. ChooseMyPlate.gov

This is a remarkably satisfying dish with a smooth texture and layered flavor. Add melon chunks or fresh berries and a slice of whole grain toast to make a nutritionally balanced meal.

Ingredients

1 tablespoon oil
6 eggs
1/2 cup non-fat milk
1/2 cup low-fat cheese, grated
1 teaspoon garlic powder
1 1/2 teaspoon oregano
Salt and pepper to taste

Directions: Preheat oven to 350°F. Put oil in a 7.5 x 3.75" loaf pan and heat in the oven for a few minutes. In a bowl, beat eggs until creamy. Mix in remaining ingredients. Pour into hot loaf pan. Bake 20 minutes or until eggs are firm. Season with salt and pepper: serve immediately. 4 eggs and 4 egg whites may be used instead of 6 eggs to reduce fat and cholesterol (nutrient analysis reflects this modification). Serves 4. Per serving: 163 calories, 13 grams protein, 11 grams fat, 3 grams carbohydrate.

DATE: _____ S M T W T F S 　　　DAILY PLANNER

APPOINTMENTS

TO DO

SCHEDULE

MEALS

B
L
D

Kaye Bailey

Kaye Bailey developed the 5 Day Pouch Test in 2007 and is the owner of LivingAfterWLS and the 5 Day Pouch Test websites. Ms. Bailey, a professional research journalist, and a bariatric RNY (gastric bypass) patient since 1999, brings professional research methodology and personal experience to her publications focused on long-lasting successful weight management after surgery.

Concerned about weight regain her bariatric surgeon advised her to "get back to basics". With that vague advice Ms. Bailey says, "I read thousands of pages and conducted interviews with medical professionals including surgeons, nutritionists, and mental health providers. I collected data from WLS post-ops who honestly and generously shared their experience. My research background gave me the methodology to collect a vast amount of data. As a patient I found answers to the questions and concerns I have in common with most patients after WLS." From that the 5DPT and related works evolved.

Kaye Bailey is the author of countless articles syndicated in several languages, and books available in print and electronic format including:

The 5 Day Pouch Test Owner's Manual

Day 6: Beyond the 5 Day Pouch Test

Cooking with Kaye Methods to Meals: Protein First Recipes

5 Day Pouch Test Complete Recipe Collection

Protein First: Understanding & Living the First Rule of WLS.

See Kaye's author page for a current catalog of all our publications. Kaye Bailey Amazon Page

She serves as Executive Editor of the LivingAfterWLS Personal Solutions journals and planners available at Amazon and the LAWLS Bookstore. The Personal Solutions planners and journals are success promoting tools for people that believe healthy living should be a simple and painless way of life.

Alphabetical Index of Recipes

1-Minute Ham and Egg Breakfast	93
Apple Folly	86
Autumn Pumpkin Oatmeal	74
Basic Microwave Coffee Cup Scramble	92
Basic Scrambled Eggs	103
Bell Pepper and Vidalia Onion Strata with Fresh Salsa	115
Berry Breakfast Parfaits	53
Breakfast Egg Spread	87
Breakfast Fruit Smoothie	29
Breakfast Tacos	105
Bulgur Porridge with Apples and Walnuts	67
California Melt	90
California Scramble	104
Cappuccino Cooler	21
Caprese Layers	86
Cheesy Baked Omelet	114
Chile Cheese Scramble	103
Chilled Coffee Protein Shake	20
Chocolate Banana Smoothie	31
Chocolate Peanut Butter Banana Smoothie	32
Chocolate Tofu Breakfast Shake	37
Cinnamon Peach Swirl	52
Cinnamon Vanilla Granola	75
Citrus Sunrise	86
Cloud Eggs	119
Confetti Scramble	109
Cottage Cheese, Egg, and Ham Muffins	53
Crème Caramel Shake	27
Denver Scramble	104
Egg, Sausage & Tomato Breakfast Bowl	95

Egg-White Whipped Vanilla Oatmeal	69
English Muffin Egg Pizzas	90
Fiesta Quesadilla	90
Ginger Yogurt with Fruit	47
Green Eggs	89
Green Smoothie from WebMD	28
Ham 'n Eggs	88
Hard Cooked Eggs	84
High Protein Coffee	21
Homestyle Scramble	104
Huevos Rancheros Scramble	105
Humble Cottage Brunch	87
Key Lime Yogurt Pie-Parfait	49
Kiwifruit-Lime Yogurt Parfait	50
Lemon-Ginger Ginseng Tea with Honey	40
Lemon-Ginger Tonic	39
Lemon-Ginger Tonic Green Tea	40
Make Ahead Breakfast Biscuit Quiches	119
Make-Ahead Breakfast Burrito	99
Mama Mia Egg Lasagna	99
Melon and Swiss Continental	87
Mocha Morning Coffee Smoothie	18
Muggy Eggs Breakfast Bar	96
Multi-Use DIY Pumpkin Spice Protein Mix	33
Oat Snack Cakes	71
Oatmeal Berry Greek Yogurt Parfait	50
Open-Face Fruit and Cheese Omelet	54
Overnight Yogurt Oatmeal: Base Recipe	73
Overnight Yogurt Oatmeal: Toppings	74
PB&J and Apple Oatmeal	71
Peanut Butter Cup Protein Shake	26
Poached Eggs over Sautéed Spinach Greens	111

Protein Pumpkin Spice Iced Coffee	35
Pumpkin Cheesecake Oatmeal	70
Pumpkin Spice Protein Coffee	35
Pumpkin Spice Protein Latte	34
Red, White, & Blue Berry Parfait	49
Salsa in the Morning Mug Scramble	95
Sausage Breakfast Muffins	114
Savory Oatmeal Egg, Turkey Bacon & Parmesan	72
Scrambled Eggs	102
Scrambled Eggs on Caramelized Onions	106
Seafood Scramble	108
Shamrock Smoothie	29
Shrimp Cocktail	86
Simple Baked Eggs	113
Simple Ginger Tonic	40
Smoked Salmon	88
Some like it Hot	89
Spicy Shakshuka	107
Spring Eggs with Salmon and Asparagus	116
Strawberry Banana Tofu Smoothie	38
Strawberry Cheesecake Shake	26
Sure to Please Baked Eggs & Cheese	120
That's a Wrap	89
The One-Pan Breakfast	110
Three-Grain Casserole	65
Tofu Tropical Green Smoothie	37
Tropical Papaya Protein Smoothie	30
Turkey Sausage Melts	91
Vegetable Quinoa	66
Veggie Egg Scramble	94

A LIVINGAFTERWLS PUBLICATION

KAYE BAILEY

Proudly serving the healthy weight management and weight loss surgery community since 2005.

COPYRIGHT © LIVINGAFTERWLS
ALL RIGHTS RESERVED

Made in the USA
Monee, IL
23 April 2020